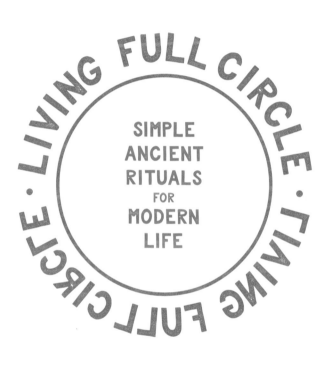

LIVING FULL CIRCLE · LIVING FULL CIRCLE ·

SIMPLE
ANCIENT
RITUALS
FOR
MODERN
LIFE

LIVING FULL CIRCLE

SIMPLE ANCIENT RITUALS FOR MODERN LIFE

Dondeena Bradley

TILLER PRESS

New York London Toronto Sydney New Delhi

TILLER PRESS

An Imprint of Simon & Schuster, Inc.
1230 Avenue of the Americas
New York, NY 10020

Copyright © 2019 by Simon & Schuster, Inc.

All rights reserved, including the right to reproduce this book or portions thereof in any form whatsoever. For information, address Simon & Schuster Subsidiary Rights Department, 1230 Avenue of the Americas, New York, NY 10020.

First Tiller Press hardcover edition December 2019

TILLER PRESS and colophon are trademarks of Simon & Schuster, Inc.

For information about special discounts for bulk purchases, please contact Simon & Schuster Special Sales at 1-866-506-1949 or business@simonandschuster.com.

The Simon & Schuster Speakers Bureau can bring authors to your live event. For more information or to book an event, contact the Simon & Schuster Speakers Bureau at 1-866-248-3049 or visit our website at www.simonspeakers.com.

Illustrations by Toby Triumph
Interior design by Jennifer Chung

Manufactured in the United States of America

10 9 8 7 6 5 4 3 2 1

Library of Congress Number: 2019947485

ISBN 978-1-9821-3296-5
ISBN 978-1-9821-3297-2 (ebook)

To our wise planet

that breathes out the sun each day

making color shine

Respect yourself and

others will respect you.

—Confucius

CONTENTS

Preface xiii

Introduction xxiii

How to Use This Book xxvii

Grounding: Connecting Body and Mind 1

 Breath IQ 4

 Breath Scan 6

 Alternate Nostril Breathing (ANB) 8

 Clean Slate 10

 Personal Spotlight: Jessica Cygan 13

 Daybreak 14

Mobilizing: "Greasing the Wheels" 17

 Joint Scan 20

 Speaking Up 22

 Belly Jump-Start 24

 Mobilizing Resilience 26

 Personal Spotlight: Nikki Calonge 28

Signaling: Gesturing Deliberate Action 29

 Self-Assurance Hand Gesture 32

 Acceptance Hand Gesture 34

 Self-Confidence Hand Gesture 36

 Grounding Hand Gesture 38

 Patience Hand Gesture 40

 Personal Spotlight: Lina Vezzani-Katano 42

Sensing: Diagnosing Hidden Barriers 43

Tongue IQ 46

Palms Up 48

Finger Tapping 50

Self-Massage 52

Warming Up 54

Personal Spotlight: Jayne Babine 57

Tranquil Shower 58

Zoning: Clearing Cluttered Space 61

Red or R-Zone 66

Orange or O-Zone 68

Yellow or Y-Zone 70

Green or G-Zone 72

Blue or B-Zone 74

Indigo or I-Zone 76

Violet or V-Zone 78

Quiet Zone 80

Good Vibe Poem 82

Re-Zone 84

Personal Spotlight: Julia Weekes 87

Judge-Free Zone 88

Shifting: Changing Things Up 91

Personal Spotlight: Daria Kalinina 93

A.M. Wake-Up Call 98

Tongue Scraping 100

Oil Pulling 102

Transitioning: Welcoming Hopeful Serendipity 105

Break | Fast 108

Preparing a Pot of *Khichdi* 110

Warm Golden Milk 112

Cumin Coriander Fennel (CCF) Tea Break 114

Silence is Golden 116

Practicing: Establishing New Routines 119

Personal Spotlight: Daria Kalinina 121

Caterpillar 122

Gratitude Journal 124

Prayer Chain 126

Private Dance Party 128

Nature Walk 130

Owning: Noticing What Flows 133

Personal Spotlight: Maryanne O'Brien 137

EMF Detox 138

Sunset Fast 140

Quick Fast 142

One-Day Fast 144

Three-Day Liver Rejuvenation 147

Detoxification Recipes 150

Basic Detox Tea 150

Liver Detox Health Drink 150

Butternut Squash Apple Soup 151

Mung Lentil Rice Soup 152

Herbal Tea (with variations) 152

Khichdi 153

Instruction—Day One 154

Instruction—Day Two 154

Instruction—Day Three 155

Spiraling: Healing Inside Outward 157

Personal Spotlight: Clarissa Lieberman 160

Glowing Skin   162

Rejuvenating Bath   164

Haiku Poem   166

Living Full Circle   169

Acknowledgments   173

Thought Bubble and

     Mastery Quote Reference Guide   175

Index   185

Journal Pages   189

PREFACE

In a fast-paced world flooded with trendy products designed to reduce stress, it's easy to get overwhelmed just trying to find simple ways to be well. However, through my own personal experience, I have come to believe that the key to sustained wellness has always been within reach through practices that have truly stood the test of time. There are hundreds of ancient rituals that help us achieve balance and wellness, yet they have been forgotten or left behind because many people think they aren't relevant anymore.

   This became my hypothesis after joining a talented group of people who were all on a path to becoming certified holistic health counselors. In this group, we welcomed people from all walks of life. We were massage therapists, fitness instructors, athletes, designers, medical professionals, yogis, dancers, scientists, electrical engineers, mothers, retirees, and financial analysts. All of us were highly credentialed in our respective fields, but we were also so much more. We were soulful, humorous, courageous, generous, humble, wise, gracious, gentle, sincere, patient, and resilient humans, who showed up to expand our knowledge of old worlds and ancient practices. We were curious about the teachings of the great seers and sages who studied the science of living a healthy and balanced life, and we all sought answers to the same question: Why does "being well" today always end up feeling like an impossible task?

I came to this group as a formally trained innovator and inventor with a master's in nutrition and a doctorate in food science who passionately believes that "stress"—both visible and hidden—is killing us and demanding that we rethink how we live our lives. Over the course of my career, I've spent decades translating science, trends, and human behaviors into new products and services in order to improve health and overall well-being. In the 1990s, I began translating health claims and nutrition profiles into more compelling nutrition labels. Twenty-five years later, translating ancient practices into a narrative for modern living was a natural and timely task to undertake. For the past fifteen years, my effort has focused on strategies for improving the lives of people living with obesity and diabetes. I became knowledgeable about these chronic conditions, and the wide gap between scientific recommendations and practical solutions. I observed time and time again that what really works is easy to say, but harder to do. By this I mean that we often think, *If I accept who I am today and commit to just one healthy practice every day, I will reach my goal.* But when it comes to acting on this commitment, we find that difficult.

The first step to fulfilling this commitment requires *accepting* who I am today. The dictionary definition of "accept" is to receive willingly, to give approval, to endure without protest, and to regard as normal. Accept me, not except me. Accept every lovely, ugly, delicious part of me. Accept how I look, what I feel, how I think, what I know, what I do not know, how I show up, what I believe, and how I choose to live my life. I pause on this idea of accepting because generally more attention is paid to picking and choosing the "one thing" to do in order to achieve the goal. This could be celery juice, a retreat, a smartphone app, a ClassPass membership, a new wardrobe. (You can probably think of a few other things that you thought were the answer to a whole new "well" life.) Glossing over acceptance held me back in the past, but unpacking it alongside changing up my daily routine has helped me soar. I call it the *real* work. Along the way, it has certainly raised a lot of questions for me, given the choices I made on my career path, my expertise, and all that I've learned from hundreds of experts in the health and wellness field over the years. Questions like: *Has wellness become a commodity at the expense of well-being?* and *Why are mental health care costs really skyrocketing?*

Let's start with the question about wellness and well-being. According to the Global Wellness Institute, there is a $4.2 trillion global wellness economy that is comprised of markets like anti-aging, beauty, wellness tourism, healthy eating, fitness, mind-body, personalized medicine, alternative medicine, and workplace wellness. Their report defines wellness as the active pursuit of choices and lifestyles that lead to a state of holistic health. Holistic health is commonly defined as a wellness approach that addresses not just the physical body but also the mental and emotional aspects of an individual. While there are thought leaders bringing forward an integrated approach to our well-being that can transform our lives, not enough is happening to ease the hectic pace of making a living, which barely allows for time to hear about new solutions, much less time to take action.

On the flip side of wellness, the rates of chronic diseases have continued to rise in the United States. According to the American Heart Association, one person in the U.S. has a stroke about every forty seconds. Moreover, not only are obesity rates not improving the way experts believe they can, but obesity-induced cancer is also on the rise. Every five years, the U.S. Departments of Agriculture (USDA) and Health and Human Services (HHS) work together to release Dietary Guidelines for Americans (DGAs), and while reducing added sugar and frequency of eating is still high on their list of preventative, "don't eat this" recommendations, my hope is that our government is moving toward providing more accessible holistic advice for all of us. After all, we know that our bodies are very much connected to our minds, and it is my belief that focusing too much on food and exercise without also acknowledging the benefits of slowing down and allowing ourselves to be more mindful in our daily lives may even factor into our society's skyrocketing mental health care costs.

Regarding these skyrocketing mental health care costs, part of the issue may be found somewhere in the space that exists between a crazy, unexpected, or tragic thing that can occur in one's life and the stark reality of having to rejoin the workplace or so-called "real life" afterward. This "in-between" space rarely gives us enough time to adequately deal with these major moments in our lives, and we are usually not well equipped to manage their impact if they turn our world upside down. The effects of floods, fatal heart attacks, overdoses, suicide, gun violence, limited cash flow, panic attacks, fires, and tragic loss are real and can be incredibly disorienting. But as a response to these events, we often self-medicate. We numb out.

I remember the "in-between" of being a few days from beginning a new job and the tragic death of my sister, Jaime. Although the company kindly suggested that I take more time before starting, I didn't trust that gesture as true as it might have been, so I began the job and slogged through the days. Fourteen months later, Konner, her daughter (my niece), passed away at age six. I remember wanting to be at the hospital with my parents and feeling disconnected from all of it. There is so much more to this story, but the point is that over a ten-year span, I have slowly shed the many layers of pain and grief that piled up as my family dealt with the twists and turns of even more pain and loss. For so long, I was in a fog and didn't know it. I can see now how I got lost in that fog because it's since lifted, and I finally feel clear again. Much of it was brought on during and after 9/11, while my own kids were quite young, and living in New York City at the time pushed me to armor up. Often, I just wanted to hide, so I buried myself in work. But unexpressed anger began leaking out of me all over the place, and I ended up battling my own demons. Ultimately, this experience allowed me to see how we put on different "faces" over our mental health, especially at the workplace. Although our society has made progress in how we manage depression, suicide, and life counseling, we desperately need to rethink and retool, given how foundational the problem really is. It will persist if we do not give it the proper care and required attention.

Have we truly forgotten what it means to care for ourselves and other human beings? In 2011, as part of a TedxOrangeCoast experience, I posed the question "How can we create a society addicted to health?" I am still wondering about that in light of all the data that shows the unintended consequences of our 24/7 habits of being "on." I wonder how we can effectively bring wellness to everyday living in ways that allow everyone to benefit, rather than just the few who have the means to pay for it. This effort should include improving the experiences around us when we are not well. Hospital experiences, in particular, shock me—not necessarily the people you encounter there, but the overall context for how a person and family experiences unexpected trauma, care, and, ideally, a path to healing. I know this is not universal, but it has been my experience. When my mom was undergoing major cancer surgery, for instance, it seemed at times that we humans were just part of the machinery. I had my own personal experience in high school, too, after spending weeks in the hospital due to a mono-induced coma. I remember lying wide awake for hours wishing that all of the piercing sounds and disgusting smells would go away. Confusing lights, disturbed sleep, crash carts rattling around creating panic. Acronyms that made no sense. And, oh, the lovely Mrs. X, who died on the other side of my curtain wall. She let out one loud, last gurgling breath that I can still hear. I was terrified. This is not how a human life should end.

With that being said, I want you to imagine yourself in the mix of that diverse group of people I described earlier who, along with myself, were studying ancient wisdom to achieve better health and be able to counsel others. In this group, we curiously immersed ourselves in hands-on learning with experts in areas such as energy management, essential oils, and color therapy. Comforting aromas of a weather-based tea recipe greeted us whenever we entered our gathering space down on Manhattan's Nassau Street. Compassionate instructors grounded us with breathwork and gentle movement. Delicious meals and mindful eating awaited us after we dissected recipes and interrogated ingredients and their sources that reflected other cultures. We observed and practiced techniques on each other, including pulse readings, tongue inspections, and touch therapy. We created a shared community of learning that far extended our time in the makeshift classroom. More than that, being a part of this group inspired us to reconsider all of those complicated, trendy, and costly wellness practices and instead "come full circle" and return to the ancient practices that still benefit us today.

Ayurveda, which literally means "the science of living," is one of these practices. Having originated in India more than five thousand years ago, it is considered to be one of the oldest healing modalities that focuses on the integration of the mind, body, and spirit. Practitioners of Ayurveda utilize all of their senses—touch, sound, sight, smell, and taste—to observe and bring the body back into balance with nature. They also hold the profound belief that we are all connected to each other as well as to our breathing planet, and they emphasize the importance of nature in our daily lives. I will never forget the full weekend of cleansing and rejuvenating I participated in with my holistic health counselor certification group, during which we placed a special focus on Ayurvedic rituals and retuning our body clocks to the natural rhythm of the sun. A fog was lifted from my head that weekend that I did not realize was there. It was not hard to remove this fog; it just required me to accept being a tad uncomfortable and to make different choices and a commitment to stay present, no matter what.

Over the course of this weekend, I experienced a number of unexpected positive benefits and personal insights. I noticed that I had been living in my head and making up stories that were not actually happening. I had no real sense of time, and I would easily disconnect from what was happening around me. Essentially, I was not fully present in my life. Now I know how it feels to be present, and that it's not okay to *not* make changes. Ultimately, being a part of this group motivated me to change up my routine and dig deeper into how I could redesign my life using the ancient rituals we studied to simply feel better every day.

Of course, a weekend of cleansing and rejuvenating is *not* a simple ritual, and I recognize that most people have busy schedules and do not have the time to slow down or the tools to intentionally focus on the state of their body-mind connection. But what I have come to believe through my group experience is that there are a number of easy ways to improve one's overall well-being using simple ancient rituals that can be done in just minutes a day. We don't need to constantly chase the "shiny new thing" or trend, only to be disappointed and disillusioned when it leaves us feeling depleted or drained. When we commit to the one small thing, and then another and another, positive change *does* happen. We don't need to overthink it; we just need to commit to it. Today I am on a mission to translate ancient practices—which at first glance may seem complicated—into easy and practical ways to jump-start care for your whole self. My goal is not to convince you of the benefits of these ancient rituals and healing techniques, but to address the bigger barriers of inertia by making them easy and worth your time to try.

I turned my holistic health counselor certification into an innovation lab. I listened, observed, and sketched concepts for easy ways to feel better. I asked classmates and colleagues about new rituals that created a tipping point for shifting their daily routine. I stripped away the foreign words to simplify the instruction. I honed in on the core component that was often overlooked and misjudged for its potential to spark positive change.

Most innovation is so obvious that we miss it, and I don't want you to miss it. By simply adding minutes-long rituals, like the ones included in this book, to your daily routine, you too can get on the path to positive change and feeling better. Stay with them long enough, and they will seep into the way you live, help you manage your emotions, and create space for the things in life that truly matter. Over time, they may even change the stories you tell yourself and how you relate to others.

Whatever fog is hanging over you will lift. You can "live full circle"—continuously coming back to you, the whole you—just like I learned to do by studying and adopting these simple ancient rituals.

INTRODUCTION

There are tons of quick and easy rituals, deeply rooted in ancient wisdom, for you to practice every day, but in this book you will find just over fifty of what I consider to be the most effective rituals, ones that require little preparation, address diverse needs, and can have a visible and positive impact, as witnessed by many of my friends and colleagues. The way in which I've organized the rituals tells its own story, which will be described in greater detail in the brief introduction to each section, and my hope is that these rituals will not only enable you to reconnect with your five senses but also improve your overall sense of self. For example, I found that adding some of the liver-cleansing and joint-care rituals into my evening routine increased my motivation to exercise, gave me more energy, and helped me bounce back more quickly after long runs or intense workouts. They also helped me become more emotionally balanced. Before I turned to studying these ancient wellness rituals, I didn't realize I was relying so much on my diet and exercise routine to obtain my personal health goals—and unintentionally leaving behind the needs of my mental and emotional state. Now I have a collection of go-to self-care practices that enhance *all* of me.

Among the rituals featured in this book are the practices of ancient Chinese qigong masters—who focused on balancing the body, mind, heart, and spirit with movement, sound healing, and visualization practices—and Ayurvedic rituals, as well as yoga and meditation breathwork and gestures that can help calm the mind, increase energy levels, and awaken our inner voice. All of these rituals are meant to help you slow down and be more present for the undoing of whatever is making you unhappy, and they will also allow your mind to become a creative force for what you need and want. My intention for sharing them with you is to provide a field guide that allows you to discover a diverse range of practices that can benefit your overall well-being. With that being said, it is not my intention to minimize the immense work that has been done by those who have devoted their lives to master and preserve these rituals and their rich history.

Finally, as a researcher, I know that developments in science distinguish our modern technology-driven world from the analog treatments of ancient times. New ideas and proofs of concepts continuously shift what we think we know, especially about how to eat or manage our health. For instance, eggs are good for you, then suddenly they are bad for you. And if eggs are turning your world upside down, then I suggest we talk. We are constantly learning and unlearning—and yet we know in our gut when something is just true. We know that resistance and negativity can undo the other supposedly good things you are doing for yourself. While it cannot always be quantified, I know that negativity is more detrimental to my health than eating less-than-healthy foods. When I was growing up, good health was simply defined as eating right, staying active, and getting plenty of sleep, probably because a lot of the rest of the good stuff was included in our everyday lives, like the positive impact of playing outdoors. Back then, I didn't understand that our body was layered with energy circuits and that simple hand gestures could enhance my energy flow, but I knew when I was in the zone.

We instinctively know that our body requires consistent care and attention, yet we need to pay as much attention to our mind and ensure it is connected to our body. I often hear people say they want tried-and-true practices, but the shiny new thing or method always seems to win out. This book is an attempt to outline the steps to these simple ancient rituals, in order to enhance aware-ness and acceptance of their possibilities and ultimately help you rethink what wellness and living holistically can be for you.

HOW TO USE THIS BOOK

Each ritual outlined in the book follows a basic format that includes a "thought bubble," a simple ancient ritual, a mastery quote, a modern take, and "Discover More," a series of suggested terms to look up if you are interested in deepening your understanding of the ritual or things and practices that are related to it.

The Format:

THOUGHT BUBBLE: *"Is anyone else thinking this but afraid to say it out loud?"*

SIMPLE ANCIENT RITUAL: A quick, step-by-step technique to try out anywhere

MASTERY QUOTE: A relevant quote to inspire your mastery of the ritual

MODERN TAKE: The insights and understanding you can glean from doing the ritual today

DISCOVER MORE: Suggested search terms

Breaking Down the Format
THOUGHT BUBBLE

The "thought bubble" for each ritual is an example that helps illustrate a need so you can better identify with the ritual. Extracting and popping these "thought bubbles" is an art—as well as critical to do—because these are the thoughts we *know* everyone is thinking but may be too hesitant to share out loud. While there could be a range of thought bubbles for every ritual, I provided one example for each in order to keep the rituals as simple and straightforward as possible. So, I encourage you to think about each thought bubble for a minute before you discount it, because there are multiple layers to probe. For example, *"I barely have enough energy to get out of bed"* could seem like an extreme statement that may not apply to you today, but we know there is a range of energy depletion that we face on certain days under different circumstances, from extreme to light, which can include *"I feel my energy flatten out as the day goes on."* That said, the rituals provided in this book are effective for any circumstance.

SIMPLE ANCIENT RITUAL

The rituals are simple, minutes-long techniques that require little to no preparation. They are derived from ancient practices and have been translated into laymen's terms. While the rituals shouldn't be thought of as quick fixes, I selected them because of their simplicity and visible impact. Following the steps for each ritual is intended to help you bring more awareness to a root cause of a particular ailment or issue you have and how to deal with it through consistent but minimal effort.

MASTERY QUOTE

Mastery begins with a simple task and proceeds by staying with it until it becomes automatic. As mundane as it may sound, I cannot stress enough the need to stick with these rituals because that is when your health and well-being will truly benefit. Be patient. Do not underestimate the power of the ritual, given the simplicity. Each mastery quote associated with a ritual is intended to make you smile and to provide inspiration that will extend the experience. My hope is that pondering on these words will help you stay on track as you customize your own daily routine of rituals that best suit your needs.

MODERN TAKE

Ancient wisdom persists and provides tools to enhance our well-being alongside the evolution of technology. The intent of the "modern take" for each ritual is to bring that wisdom back into view so that it can coexist alongside present-day things like your wearable technology or current exercise routine. In other words, this section pulls out the nugget of ancient wisdom from each ritual and applies it to our modern lives.

DISCOVER MORE

A journey to better self-care is different for each of us. There is a wealth of information to discover about feeling better and your own personal well-being, including breathwork, energy management, shifting your mind-set, cleanses, and other related topics. In stripping down the ritual to its core for easy integration into your life, there may be specific rituals that you want to learn more about or dig deeper into, so check out the "Discover More" terms associated with each ritual to help you get started.

What You Need

This book is a guide for you to use at any moment, but you might find yourself wanting a few things at your side when doing these rituals. When I practice them, I typically prefer to seek out a quiet spot, where I can stretch out on a mat while jotting down my thoughts in a journal. (There are also journal pages in the back of this book for you to use at your leisure.) I also like to have my thermos handy for a sip of warm water or steeped tea when I want it.

For a few rituals, you will need to purchase a jar of refined organic coconut oil or a box of individual packets. Coconut oil is a solid base to use for oil pulling or self-massage. As you practice self-massage, you may find that you want to expand your tools and use other oils matched to your dosha (e.g. sesame oil), essential oils, dried spices and seeds for pastes, or certain teas. I dedicated a couple of shelves in a kitchen cabinet to organizing things like oils, seeds, turmeric, basmati rice, lentils, and ghee, but this is not required to get started. Customizing the rituals to my own likes and dislikes was helpful for me to learn more about them—and made practicing even more fun.

Finally, a special section guides you through a three-day liver rejuvenation, which includes various recipes to detoxify and cleanse your liver as well as clear out your energy zones. Check out the recipes and order any specialty ingredients in advance of scheduling a time you can commit to it. This three-day rejuvenation had surprising results for me and my colleagues, so I encourage you to adapt it in whatever way works for you. There are benefits to taking the time to nourish our overworked bodies—especially during a change of season.

Personal Spotlights

Dispersed throughout the book, you will find a collection of "personal spotlights." These are insights from some of my colleagues in the holistic health counselor certification group and a few others who have undergone similar certification coursework, and their stories are intended to highlight the unexpected impact of adopting new rituals into your daily routine.

I cannot say enough how insignificant we thought some of these rituals would be before we started doing them, yet sharing our personal transformations with one another motivated us all to stick with them. I am honored to include a brief glimpse into the practices and their experiences in order to demonstrate the great impact that a tiny change can have on many areas of our lives. Being surrounded by colleagues who became my teachers and mentors was an extraordinary gift as I began rethinking my philosophy and dismantling the structure of my day-to-day life. It allowed me to deal with extraordinary change and personal challenge in healthier ways, and for that I am forever grateful.

Ritual Themes

The fifty rituals are curated into thematic sections in order to anchor you to an overarching narrative about spiraling up and ultimately feeling better. There are ten themes in total starting with grounding, and each bundle of rituals serves as an individual step toward taking ownership of your own well-being. Practicing them with the theme in mind will provide insight into areas where you soar or where you get stuck. For instance, if you tend to signal action yet never quite transition into a new phase, it may be time for you to evaluate the hidden barriers that are holding you back.

Notice the stories you tell yourself and jot them down as you work your way through the ritual themes.

Ten Themes of the Ancient Rituals
Grounding: Connecting Body and Mind
Mobilizing: "Greasing the Wheels"
Signaling: Gesturing Deliberate Action
Sensing: Diagnosing Hidden Barriers
Zoning: Clearing Cluttered Space
Shifting: Changing Things Up
Transitioning: Welcoming Hopeful Serendipity
Practicing: Establishing New Routines
Owning: Noticing What Flows
Spiraling: Healing Inside Outward

Now it's time to dive in and uncover ways to reduce stress and rebalance yourself beyond just eating better and exercising. Keep in mind that stress comes in many forms, including psychological, so listen for your own excuses and take on the challenge of creating a new reality of choosing to feel good. And most of all, please be patient with yourself. As my wise teacher would often say—patience protects the body and the mind.

GROUNDING

CONNECTING BODY AND MIND

CONNECTING THE BODY to the mind or the mind to the body equals grounding. Breath is the bridge that links the two, yet we often overlook the power of the breath, especially the deeper breath, when we are under stress. Extreme stress, such as those feelings experienced after the loss of a job or an unexpected death of a family member, hurts deeply. Over time, it takes a toll on how we can show up for ourselves and for others. Too much stress can literally and figuratively hurt and harden the heart. Do not let it.

Think about it this way: Your brain gives your body direction for handling stress. Stress hits, and one part of your nervous system tells the heart to pump faster. Another part calms the heart back down. And another system, called the limbic system, manages the emotional responses—from angry or fearful to happy or calm. Constant stress makes it harder for the brain to coordinate all of this information you need, and while this may be an oversimplification, missteps in how the body communicates does not have the intended effect.

Adequately handling stress is essential, and breath is an underutilized partner. Breath is healing. Taking a deep breath activates the nerves that enable the ability to calm down. While breath works hard on its own, it shows up more effectively when it is intentionally directed. Increasing the awareness of breath and noticing the control of it—how deep, how shallow, how fast, how slow, even how cold or how hot—is vital to well-being. In yoga, a formal practice of controlling the breath, also known as *pranayama*, can be broken down into three parts: taking breath in, holding it, and releasing it. Focusing on all three parts, or the "breathwork," is beneficial for maintaining balance when dealing with stressors throughout the day.

The following rituals are so simple that their impact may be underestimated. One ritual is simply paying attention to and noticing the breath. Another ritual, alternate nostril breathing (or ANB), releases anxiety very quickly, especially in high-stress situations. Doing this particular ritual may feel weird at first, but once you experience its benefits, I'm certain it will become a go-to for finding calm in chaotic circumstances and improving your emotional resilience. All in all, acknowledging and leveraging breath is vital and a great place for your full-circle wellness journey to start.

BREATH IQ

THOUGHT BUBBLE:
"There are so many distractions, I cannot focus!"

SIMPLE ANCIENT RITUAL:
- Sit or lie down in a comfortable position.
- Notice your breath.
- Follow it in and out of your nose.
- Notice the pace, the depth, and the temperature.
- As it comes in, note your belly gently expanding.
- Feel yourself settle with each breath.
- Repeat throughout the day.

MASTERY QUOTE:
"When the breath is still, so is the mind."
—*The* Hatha Yoga Pradīpikā

MODERN TAKE:

How we breathe is important. Breathwork helps us focus, especially when our days are full and overscheduled. Demands from our work, family, and even financial pressures tend to distract us from pausing to take two minutes for breathwork. As a result, our breath can be fast and shallow. The use of only a fraction of our lungs results in an imbalance of the oxygen that charges us and the carbon dioxide that clears away the toxic wastes from our body. A breath regimen helps cleanse the body and the mind.

DISCOVER MORE:

pranayama; meditation; breath control; breath sensing; breathing exercises

BREATH SCAN

THOUGHT BUBBLE:

"What is the correct way to breathe—through my nose or my mouth?"

SIMPLE ANCIENT RITUAL:

- Sit or lie down in a comfortable position.
- Take two minutes and notice your breath.
- Breathe through your nose, not your mouth, and keep your mouth closed.
- Let your belly expand as air flows in and release as air flows out.
- If your breath is rough or uneven, stop and relax.
- As you breathe in and out, count each breath cycle.
- If you become distracted, begin the counting again.
- Set a goal to breathe through ten cycles that are smooth and steady.

MASTERY QUOTE:

"Great things are done by a series of small things brought together."
—Vincent van Gogh

MODERN TAKE:

It seems foolish to think that we need to be taught how to properly breathe. Yet, as you increase your own breath IQ, you may notice that your breath has become modified and restricted. The nose is equipped to keep out impurities and cold air. It has built-in defense mechanisms, such as a screen of tiny hairs that trap dust along with a long, winding passage that is lined to warm up cool air. The sense of smell detects poisonous gas or toxic mold that may injure your health. Notice if you breathe too much through your mouth, and shift by closing your mouth.

DISCOVER MORE:

prana; healthy breathing; *bastrika*; breathing process; focus; *Savasana*; breath meditation

ALTERNATE NOSTRIL BREATHING (ANB)

THOUGHT BUBBLE:

"I can hardly breathe. I feel panicky."

SIMPLE ANCIENT RITUAL:

- Starting with your right nostril, take your thumb and ring finger and block the nostril while keeping your mouth closed. Then breathe in via the left nostril.
- Hold the breath and then close off the left nostril.
- Exhale through the right nostril.
- Breathe in via the right nostril, and then close off the right nostril.
- Exhale through the left nostril.
- Inhale through the left nostril, and then close off the left nostril.
- Exhale through the right nostril.
- Repeat the rotation three times or until you feel calm.

MASTERY QUOTE:

*"If we take care of the minutes,
the years will take care of themselves."*
—Benjamin Franklin

MODERN TAKE:

Breath can be modified or restricted due to subconsciously slouching, sitting for long hours, or even being so focused on what is in front of you that the breath becomes erratic. So pay attention to these barriers to better breathing and schedule time for breathwork. Notice how emotions change the way we breathe. When we feel fear, anxiety, or panic, our breathing accelerates. Give yourself time to breathe through these emotions. It will pay in dividends. ANB is a deliberate practice, allowing for visualizing the breath as it moves from one side of the body to the other with intention. It can also balance our masculine and feminine energies within the body while calming that panicky feeling.

DISCOVER MORE:

Nadi Shodhana; P300; cognitive processes; nasal breathing; *dirgha* breath

CLEAN SLATE

THOUGHT BUBBLE:

"I have too much on my plate, and the day hasn't even started!"

SIMPLE ANCIENT RITUAL:

- Set an alarm for five minutes from now.
- Sit in a comfortable posture with your spine erect.
- Quiet your mind, and notice your breath.
- Begin by inhaling deeply, and internally say the word "So."
- As you exhale completely, say to yourself, "Hum."
- Follow the breath in and out of the nose, and continue to repeat "So . . . Hum."
- Do this practice every morning.
- Extend the practice to ten minutes when possible.

MASTERY QUOTE:

"Poetry is breathing words that give a reader pause."
—Ankita Singhal

MODERN TAKE:

Practicing this ritual helps clear the mind, so throughout the rest of the day there is a steady calm to help us process information better, stay relaxed, and make clear-minded decisions. This is a steady, in-and-out breathing technique. This practice of intentionally saying the same words over and over gives the mind something to hold on to so it can stay focused on the ritual. This warming breath is especially good for bringing a cool body into balance.

DISCOVER MORE:

chanting; mantras, transcendental meditation; mindfulness; vedic chanting

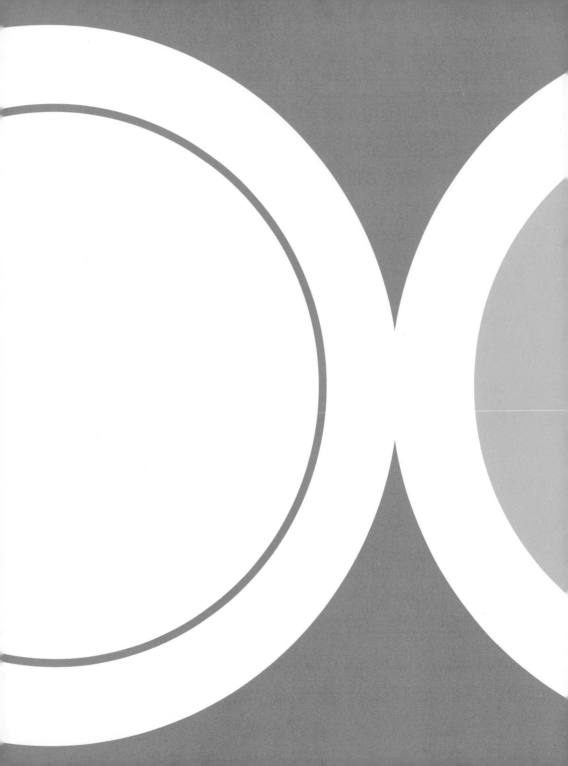

JESSICA CYGAN

I am a finance professional as well as a student and teacher of yoga and Ayurveda. Mornings are very special to me, and so I make it a priority to spend quiet time greeting each new day. I've always believed in natural remedies to maintain health. Nature provides all that the body needs—as well as the mind. A friend recommended a book that introduced the ancient practices of Ayurveda, and from there I was hooked. Learning about these easy and often overlooked techniques has provided me with a wealth of knowledge, which is now intuitive. This has empowered me to go deeper in my exploration of breathwork and its role in the body-mind connection. I wake up early every morning and begin with prayer, gentle stretching, and, if nature allows, a run in the park. Next are breakfast and coffee, where I mindfully am present for the meal in front of me. Then it is "go time," and I am off to work. I am steadily building a deeper awareness of my breath and its power to help me stay fully present throughout the day (see Breath Scan, page 6). My consistency is key to strengthening my abilities through daily meditation, breathwork, and subtle yoga postures. The breath is the manifestation of my vital life force, which I can inconspicuously manage throughout the day.

DAYBREAK

THOUGHT BUBBLE:
"I need some peace and quiet in my life."

SIMPLE ANCIENT RITUAL:
- Wake up a bit earlier at the same time every day (e.g., sunrise).
- Make a list of concerns that you want to release.
- Engage in a routine of gentle stretching.
- Drink your coffee and/or eat your breakfast quietly.
- Use the extra time to enable yourself to reach a personal goal.

MASTERY QUOTE:
"It is well to be up before daybreak, for such habits contribute to health, wealth, and wisdom."
—Aristotle

MODERN TAKE:

Do you start your day by pressing the snooze button so you can get ten more minutes of sleep? Try starting your day with the sunrise. It will help you focus on yourself and the needs of the day without interruption. Keeping your body on a sleep routine makes it easier to wake up naturally. Reward yourself in the morning with gentle stretching. Breathwork will set the tone for the entire day. It is a mind-set. All it requires is attention; follow the breath, and notice how it moves with and within the body. Bringing awareness to the breath has heightened my appreciation for all the body does on its own, without my intervening.

DISCOVER MORE:

pranayama; Nadi Shodhana; mindfulness; breathing exercises; mindful morning routine

MOBILIZING

"GREASING THE WHEELS"

MOTION AND MOVEMENT are different, yet equally important. Do all of your toes and fingers have their full range of motion? Over time, you lose flexibility if you are not intentional about creating a daily motion routine beyond getting your steps in with a walk or a run. More than 30 million Americans suffer from arthritis, and two-thirds are of working age (18 to 65+). So, even if you miss out on your walk or run, including circular rotation of your joints while sitting or getting ready for bed is beneficial.

The motion of all your internal parts that keep you on track throughout the day is important, too. For instance, gentle waves of motion prevent constipation, which can be caused by sitting too long, dietary changes, and dehydration. The inside of our body relies on motion to pump blood through our circulatory system, breathe air down and back out of our lungs, and move food through more than twenty feet of a coiled digestive track. Rubbing your stomach in a circular motion can help move things along. Soaking in a hot tub of water helps the circulation of blood throughout your body. Even drinking hot water, perhaps surprisingly, has a similar effect. As you raise your internal body temperature, you start to sweat, which is essential to getting rid of toxins. The following rituals focus on increasing circular motion on the outside and inside of the body in order to mobilize your energy, directly and indirectly.

JOINT SCAN

THOUGHT BUBBLE:

"My stiff fingers and knees keep me from doing things I enjoy."

SIMPLE ANCIENT RITUAL:

- Scan your toes, feet, ankles, knees, hips, lower back, shoulders, wrists, neck, and jaw.
- Notice if they move easily.
- Do they crackle and pop when you move them?
- Do any of your fingers lock up?
- Use a light oil, like coconut oil, and gently massage it into your joints before bed.

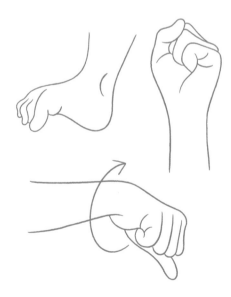

"Little by little, one travels far."
—Spanish proverb

MODERN TAKE:

A stiff neck or stiff fingers, knees, or ankles can be barriers when you want to get into the flow of your day. Poor posture that results from using the computer for long hours or even sleeping in an uncomfortable position can take their toll. Straining during a quick exercise routine can make you feel even worse. Gentle stretching, self-massage, and applying moist heat can help relax tight muscles. A daily routine of gentle massage on areas needing the most attention will increase mobility over time.

DISCOVER MORE:

self-massage; circulation; body oils; joint health; foam rollers; essential oils

SPEAKING UP

THOUGHT BUBBLE:
"Why don't I just say something?"

SIMPLE ANCIENT RITUAL:
- Pretend you are about to give the most important speech of your life.
- Say your full name out loud: "I am . . ."
- Repeat this five times.
- Notice if your voice is shaky or clear; high or low; flat or full of expression.
- Keep saying this until your voice sounds like a leader you would follow.

MASTERY QUOTE:
"There is no greater agony than bearing an untold story inside you."
—Maya Angelou

MODERN TAKE:

Mobilizing your voice takes practice. It might be difficult at first, but expressing yourself openly and honestly will make you feel like a weight has been lifted off your shoulders. Saying your name with courage is part of leading with conviction. There is no right or wrong way of expressing yourself, but ensuring that you are heard without being overbearing will enable better communication with others. The tone and confidence in your voice is an indicator of your readiness to tell your story and to take a stand when needed.

DISCOVER MORE:

Kirtan; speech therapy; Meisner technique; public speaking; throat chakra

BELLY JUMP-START

THOUGHT BUBBLE:
"I sit most of the day and cannot stay regular!"

SIMPLE ANCIENT RITUAL:
- Start the day with a glass of warm water to enhance the urge to evacuate your bowel.
- Place your palm on your abdomen.
- Make a small, circular, clockwise motion around the belly button.
- Widen the circle until you cover the entire belly.
- Repeat 5-10 times to help increase flow in your digestive track.

MASTERY QUOTE:
"I've had it with you and your emotional constipation."
—Washington Irving

MODERN TAKE:

Yes, we experience both physical and emotional constipation. Knowing our body inside and out helps us pay more attention to our needs. Learn where your organs are located, especially in your abdominal cavity, and give them an occasional massage. Increasing blood flow to your liver or helping the flow of digested food through your intestines may be needed during inactive times of your life. Before modern plumbing, our ancestors emptied the bowel using a muscle that is activated by squatting. The design of the modern toilet is flawed and can make it even more physically challenging to enable a bowel movement, but regular elimination is important for good health. Paying attention to the texture and temperature of the nourishment you put into your mouth can make a big difference in your ability to maintain a regular routine.

DISCOVER MORE:

visceral massage; poop button; constipation; puborectalis muscle; yoga for digestion; stomach massage; digestive health

THOUGHT BUBBLE:

"My feet are tired and hurt after a long day."

SIMPLE ANCIENT RITUAL:

- Before bed, massage your feet with oil (e.g., coconut oil).
- Start with the heel and massage its padding.
- Move next to the outer blade of the foot.
- Next, gently massage each toe and the pads of skin underneath each.
- End by massaging the inner arch.
- After finishing, thank your feet and say, "I propel forward with resilience."

MASTERY QUOTE:

"At the end of the day, let there be no excuses, no explanations, no regrets."
—Steve Maraboli

MODERN TAKE:

Taking care of the feet is very important to maintain mobility. Ancient gurus even mapped energy channels from specific areas on the foot to corresponding internal organs and would massage these areas to help relieve tension throughout the body (a practice that came to be known as reflexology). Be kind to your feet by keeping them clean and wearing comfortable shoes and socks. Keep a tennis ball handy, and roll it over your feet to help strengthen the muscles and improve flexibility of the joints.

DISCOVER MORE:

dosha type; acupuncture; aikido; pressure points; foot chakras; foot massage; reflexology

NIKKI CALONGE

I am a student of yoga, aikido, and dance/movement therapy. Each morning, I practice yoga and sit to meditate, and then I teach a session or take class at my dojo. When I'm not teaching, I'm in rehearsal for theater and dance; live performance is important to my creative life. I stay curious to learn how to care for myself and others in a way that is natural, clear, and holistic.

In the evening, I massage my feet and consciously thank them for all the hard work they do (see Mobilizing Resilience, page 26). I mentally refer to the Ayurveda foot map and start with the heel and its padding, which takes the most impact, especially for the stubborn and ambitious. Then I move to the lateral arch (outer blade) that is an energy channel to help keep the spine strong and supple. The toes and mounds underneath the foot get lots of attention so that the five senses and organs they are connected to maintain their vitality and responsiveness. The medial arch (inner arch) of the foot is last; it is where the soul resides. This dome is designed to propel us forward with resilience. Taking care of my feet every evening is a way to reflect on how I carry myself through the day. It relieves tension and makes me notice the way the body bears itself. My hands and feet feel the tiny shifts of attitude and perspective that accumulate over time, as I remember that real change doesn't always happen at once.

SIGNALING

GESTURING DELIBERATE ACTION

OUR BODY LANGUAGE speaks volumes in terms of how we communicate what we feel. We talk with our hands—whether we make an angry gesture when someone cuts us off while we're driving or a hand motion that emphasizes a particular comment. There are one hundred or so intentional hand gestures, called mudras, that are found in ancient practices and are go-tos when it comes to shifting your energy and overall mood. While some have been used for spiritual practices, many have been leveraged to improve the physical condition. In this way, hand gestures have emerged as a field of science, in which each finger represents a fundamental element in the body. When the fingers are positioned in certain ways, it is believed that we can influence the flow of energy in the body.

Self-awareness of my feelings and motives has drastically changed since I have become more vigilant about incorporating ancient rituals in order to maintain an even, positive attitude throughout the day. If I encounter an intense conversation and notice my body is having a visceral reaction, for instance, I rely on a hand gesture to ground me without anyone noticing. This practice enables me to observe what is actually happening without pulling me into unnecessary negative interactions. Practicing different hand gestures is also a great opportunity to stretch and work the fingers while enhancing the mobility of the joints. I encourage you to stick with these practices, as there are many layers to them— and, in turn, many benefits to reap over time.

SELF-ASSURANCE HAND GESTURE

THOUGHT BUBBLE:

"Why do I keep second-guessing myself? I know I can do it."

SIMPLE ANCIENT RITUAL:

- Hold up all five fingers on one hand.
- Touch the tips of your thumb and ring finger.
- Keep the other fingers relaxed.
- Hold this gesture for at least 2–3 minutes.
- Repeat throughout the rest of the day.

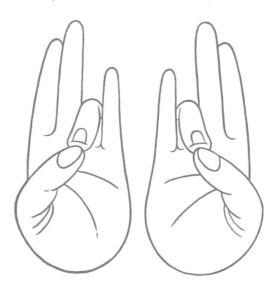

"They are not exercises, but techniques which place the physical body in positions that cultivate awareness, relaxation, concentration, and meditation."
—Swami Satyananda Saraswati

MODERN TAKE:

Who doesn't need a little pick-me-up throughout the day? This hand gesture increases stability and enhances self-assurance. I know that when I am in my zone, I feel like I can accomplish just about anything. Use this as a boost to remind yourself that everything you need is inside of you. Mudras are an effective way to move energy throughout the body. Gurus advise doing the gestures several times a day for a few minutes, so try this the next time you are walking to a meeting or standing in a line.

DISCOVER MORE:

prithvi mudra; yoga mudras; meditation; *pranayama*

ACCEPTANCE HAND GESTURE

THOUGHT BUBBLE:

"I feel really sad and cannot seem to shake it."

SIMPLE ANCIENT RITUAL:

- Hold up all five fingers on one hand.
- Fold the index finger into the space between the thumb and the index finger.
- Allow the index fingernail to touch the fold of skin between thumb and index finger.
- Join the nail of the thumb with the nail of the little finger.
- Hold in place for at least 2–3 minutes.
- Repeat throughout the rest of the day.

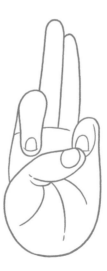

"Acceptance doesn't mean resignation; it means understanding that something is what it is and that there's got to be a way through it."
—Michael J. Fox

MODERN TAKE:

Practicing the acceptance hand gesture has become intuitive to combat those reappearing voices of protest and accepting me as I am today. Not fully accepting how I look, what I feel, how I think, what I know, or what I believe has held me back or certainly bottled me up. This mudra is intended to help bring about a mood of acceptance to overcome sadness or unnecessary resistance to uncomfortable situations. As I have reflected on choices or the loss of my sister, "acceptance" for what is has been a lesson that shows up over and over again. On hard days full of intense sadness, it would not be uncommon for me to hold the gesture for fifteen minutes or make it a part of my morning routine before I set out on my day. Don't gloss over acceptance.

DISCOVER MORE:

mudra; yoga mudras; meditation; *pranayama*

SELF-CONFIDENCE
HAND GESTURE

THOUGHT BUBBLE:

"I am tired of holding back and not speaking up."

SIMPLE ANCIENT RITUAL:

- Hold up all five fingers on both hands.
- Bend your index fingers slightly, almost 90 degrees from the top of your middle fingers.
- Rest the upper pad of your thumbs on the side of your index fingers, just below the nail.
- Keep the other fingers straight.
- Hold in place for at least 2–3 minutes.
- Repeat throughout the rest of the day.

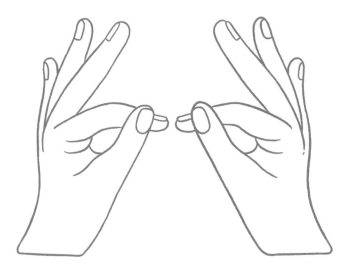

MODERN TAKE:

Self-confidence is key to accomplishing your goals because it is really about trusting yourself. I can trust myself because I know and accept who I am. I understand me. This self-awareness of feelings, beliefs, and behaviors are clues that lead to even more self-confidence in keeping fear or anxiety at bay when you know you want to show up for yourself. Developing heightened self-awareness takes time and can be deepened by adding simple hand gestures into your response to what is happening in the moment.

DISCOVER MORE:

ahamkara mudra; yoga mudras; meditation; chakra; *pranayama*

GROUNDING HAND GESTURE

THOUGHT BUBBLE:

"I feel so frenzied and just need to get a grip."

SIMPLE ANCIENT RITUAL:

- Hold up all five fingers on one hand.
- Touch the tips of your thumb and index finger.
- Keep your other fingers straight, but relaxed.
- Hold in place for at least 2–3 minutes.
- Repeat throughout the rest of the day.

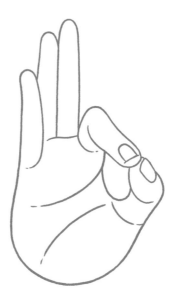

MASTERY QUOTE:

*"All the art of living lies in a fine mingling of
letting go and holding on."*
—Henry Havelock Ellis

MODERN TAKE:

Grounding helps you feel more balanced and allows energy to better flow throughout your body. Pay attention to the many factors that affect being in balance. When you are out of balance, you can be prone to swelling, sinus headaches, sore throats, constipation, insomnia, and other ailments that signal that part of you is out of balance. An Ayurveda specialist would determine your *dosha* type (or the levels of the five elements that you are comprised of) and identify ways to bring you back into balance. I notice that a natural smile emerges as I take the time to ground and come into balance.

DISCOVER MORE:

gyan mudra; yoga mudras; meditation; *pranayama*; *dosha* type

PATIENCE HAND GESTURE

THOUGHT BUBBLE:

"I am so sleep deprived, I am easily triggered and upset."

SIMPLE ANCIENT RITUAL:

- Hold up all five fingers on one hand.
- Touch the tips of your thumb and middle finger.
- Keep the other fingers relaxed.
- Hold in place for at least 2–3 minutes.
- Repeat throughout the rest of the day.

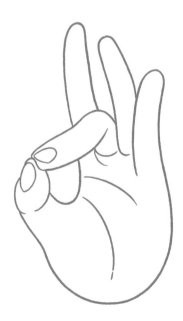

MODERN TAKE:

When are you most likely to lose your patience? Is it when your plans are interrupted during an overly scheduled day? I generally lose my patience when I am sleep deprived and overwhelmed by the long list of things needing my attention. Whatever triggers you, stop and take a couple minutes to bring awareness to the need for patience. Take a few slow, deep breaths to help calm the mind and body. It may prevent mistakes that take even more time to correct.

DISCOVER MORE:

shuni mudra; patience; yoga mudras; meditation; *pranayama*

LINA VEZZANI-KATANO

I am an energetic, twenty-nine-year-old female who trains thirteen hours per week for boxing. I'm also certified as a holistic practitioner and am taking an online course to become a UX (user experience) designer. I practice yoga and meditation and am stitching it all together to see a whole picture of what health can be for me.

I started boxing because I felt stuck in my life—stagnant, frustrated, and unchallenged. Boxing training requires intense focus—[and] my day is structured with rituals to reach my goals. [But] I get called-out by my coaches for "jumping" while I am sparring because they see that I am not grounding myself. Without "rooting" my feet into the ring floor, I lose my balance, which translates into a fall from an unexpected blow, losing full strength in my punch, or being unable to dodge punches given that I deplete my energy more quickly. Boxing is a mental sport, so I must summon my full focus on demand and sustain it. That can be challenging if I am not taking care of my whole body, and sometimes focus is hard to summon immediately on cue. Therefore, focusing on the basics, gesturing with my feet and hands (see Patience Hand Gesture, page 40), and recharging my root energy are key.

SENSING

DIAGNOSING HIDDEN BARRIERS

SENSING IS VITAL for well-being. Evaluating your own self-care from a multi-sensorial point of view will inspire you to enhance your approach and, over time, help you experience surprising results. When doing these rituals, all of my senses have a say—touch, sight, smell, sound, and taste—and introduce me to all sorts of things that help me feel better. I now rely on self-massage to recharge my ankles after a long run or my knuckles, "undoing" all the time spent typing on the computer. Colors in my wardrobe lift my mood. Obsidian, jade, or even heart-shaped stones that I have collected on nature walks are placed in my pocket to help shift my self-talk when a moment does not unfold as planned. After my sister died, rubbing that stone in my pocket helped me stay present when disorienting memories would pop into my mind. Listening to different genres of music, including the sounds of nature, help me pivot and shift my mind-set from the hectic pace and loud noises of New York City to winding down for the night. I use a diffuser to disperse essential oils throughout stale air—such as sweet orange, lemongrass, or rosemary to help motivate, purify, or focus me, respectively, and rejuvenate me while I work. A drop of lavender oil on my pillowcase signals my body that it's time to go to sleep. Sensing introduced me to so many different ways of holistic self-care, and it keeps me more balanced.

Our individual body parts need a break, and because we do not see their inner workings, we often forget about the demands we place on them. Our skin helps protect against bacteria, viruses, and other harmful substances in the environment, but a daily self-massage will lubricate, nourish, and enable it to do its job better. If we shower constantly and do not recharge our skin, it cannot as effectively protect us. Our liver never rests if we constantly graze, and that can affect our energy level. When tiredness finally sets in, relying on caffeine may also not be the best answer. Actually, cleaning and clearing out the liver can help us smooth out the inconsistencies in our energy levels without relying on external solutions. We do not necessarily see our liver, but we can lay our hands on our largest internal organ and actually feel it throbbing when it is overworked. It is located in the upper right portion of the abdomen beneath the diaphragm and below the stomach. Our stomach is located on the upper left side and creates a smoothie out of the food and beverages we put into our mouth while maintaining the optimal pH. If we constantly drink ice-cold water while we eat, we affect the function of our stomach and its ability to efficiently prepare food for digestion. A solid night of sleep rejuvenates our brain and nervous system, so sleep is not just about the number of hours we rest. Depression, for instance, can cause us to sleep more than we actually need, therefore not giving our body the jump-start it should have at the beginning of the day.

Ultimately, nurturing yourself through both motion and movement, inside and out, can increase your understanding of what your body needs. So explore ways of self-care using the five senses and increase your sense making.

TONGUE IQ

THOUGHT BUBBLE:

"My tongue feels thick. Yuck!"

SIMPLE ANCIENT RITUAL:

- Look at your tongue in the mirror every day.
- Notice if there are any changes in color, texture, coating, and the taste buds.
- Is your tongue moist or dry? If it's dry, your body may be dehydrated.
- Is the color predominantly red? There may be excess acid in your stomach.
- Is the tongue coated? Food may not have not broken down enough to move down the digestive tract.

MASTERY QUOTE:

"The body never lies." —Mae West

MODERN TAKE:

In Ayurveda, practitioners use a tongue evaluation to assess the state of a person's health. The tongue is the beginning of the digestive tract, as well as a surface that is a map of the body—just like our hands and feet—so it can help identify imbalances we may have. For example, *ama*, in Ayurveda, is the accumulation of improperly digested food and toxins that build up in the digestive tract, which in turn causes a coating on the tongue. Using a tongue scraper every morning can help remove this coating. A white, thick creamy residue on the scraper indicates carbohydrate-rich food or drink that did not get fully digested before bedtime. It is also a sign to eat lighter and incorporate more vegetables and fruits into your diet throughout the next day.

DISCOVER MORE:

tongue cleaner; *ama*; cracked tongue; taste buds; tongue scraping; oral hygiene; bad breath; ayurvedic tongue map

PALMS UP

THOUGHT BUBBLE:

"Another deep breath? I think I am going to lose it!"

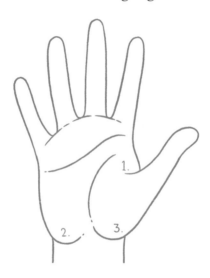

SIMPLE ANCIENT RITUAL:

- Hold out your hand with your palm facing up.
- Use your index finger and thumb to apply gentle pressure on each point called out in the illustration.
- Hold each point for a count of three.
- Cycle through each point three times.
- Press on the meaty point of the hand between the index finger and thumb.
- Press on the spot below the pinky finger where the palm meets the wrist.

- Press on the spot below the thumb where the palm meets the wrist.
- Alternate hands.

MASTERY QUOTE:

"When anger arises, think of the consequences."
—Confucius

MODERN TAKE:

As with traditional acupuncture needles, applying pressure to specific places on the body can relieve tension and pain. The body is a grid of energy points and circuits that respond to massage and pressure, and Ayurveda identifies more than one hundred energy points throughout the body that are physically located over the lymph nodes and at the joints where bone, ligaments, muscle, nerves, and blood vessels intersect. Knowing where to apply pressure in order to relieve tension is handy if you find yourself in a stressful or high-pressure situation. I especially rely on pressure points when I travel, am enduring a very long conference call, or need to stay engaged in a business meeting. It is helpful to become familiar with your pressure points.

DISCOVER MORE:

acupuncture; reflexology; pressure points; hand map; acupressure; *marma* therapy

FINGER TAPPING

THOUGHT BUBBLE:

"The pain is so bad; I am desperate for relief."

SIMPLE ANCIENT RITUAL:

- Identify a pain in your body.
- Label the emotion you feel.
- Give it an intensity score from 1 to 10, with 10 being the highest.
- Make this statement: "I acknowledge this pain and accept myself."
- Tap at least five times on the spot while making the statement.
- Now tap five times on each point shown on the diagram while making the statement.

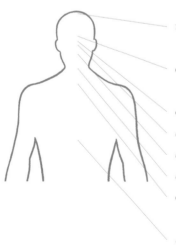

top of head: tap with all fingers in the middle

eyebrow: tap at the start of the brow near the nose

outer eye: tap near the temple

under eye: tap above cheekbone

under nose: tap above lip

under chin: tap near slight indentation

collarbone: tap underneath collarbone close to the sternum

under arm: tap about 4 inches down

*"The latest research has shown when we tap on
the endpoints of meridians in the body,
we send a calming signal to the amygdala
(the fight-or-flight center) in the brain."
—Nick Ortner, from an interview with
The Connecticut Post (May 25, 2013)*

MODERN TAKE:

Tapping is a practice derived from the ancient mapping of our body energy. With this simple technique, you use your fingers to lightly tap on specific areas of your body to amplify a signal to your brain. Simple touch can create a sensation that generates a powerful and positive wave of emotion. The skin is the largest organ in your body, and every inch contains a network of nerves that support and protect you. The skin is like an electric system; it requires care and protection to allow the current to flow.

DISCOVER MORE:

marmas; tapping; meridians; acupuncture; acupressure; *prana*

SELF-MASSAGE

THOUGHT BUBBLE:

"My neck is stiff, and my jaw feels tight."

SIMPLE ANCIENT RITUAL:

- Place 1 teaspoon of warm coconut oil on the tips of your middle and ring fingers.
- Apply the oil to your collarbone, moving upward to the chin, cheeks, face, and forehead.
- Apply around the eyes, gently moving in a clockwise direction.
- Repeat this process five times.
- Apply 1 tablespoon of warm coconut oil to the scalp.
- Place all five fingers on the hairline of your forehead.
- Slightly tap, moving from your hairline toward the back of your head.
- Continuously apply pressure, repeating front to back 10 times.

MASTERY QUOTE:

"A gentle touch is all it takes to tame the wildest of men."
—Anthony T. Hincks

MODERN TAKE:

Touch is essential to holistic health, and self-massage both increases blood flow and soothes the nervous system. In the Ayurveda tradition, there are 108 specific energy points on the human body; called *marmas*, these energy points are extremely sensitive and important for maintaining balance, so start building a daily ritual for a self-massage so you can begin activating these points. Any time of day works for self-massage, but try to do it when you are not rushed and can take the time to enjoy it.

DISCOVER MORE:

abhyanga; lymph drainage; *marmas*; aromatherapy; essential oils; ayurvedic medicine; mineral oils

WARMING UP

THOUGHT BUBBLE:

"I feel so cold; I can't warm up."

SIMPLE ANCIENT RITUAL:

- Add a few drops of lavender oil to a quarter cup of coconut oil.
- Gently massage your hands and feet.

OR

- Place a drop of thyme or clove oil onto the skin of your forearm.
- Warmth will emerge within 15 minutes.

MASTERY QUOTE:

"There is no illusion greater than fear."

—Lao Tzu, Tao Te Ching

MODERN TAKE:

Aromas can either fire us up or help us calm down based on what is physically and mentally happening within us, and aromatherapy is the use of aromatic essential oils found in nature in order to benefit our mood and even protect our health. Most items in your kitchen pantry or refrigerator have an aroma that affects you. The smell of cinnamon can bring back memories of a meal with a loved one. The nauseating smell of sour meat or milk sends the message "Do not eat or drink this or you will become ill." Pay attention to your personal reaction to the scents of your favorite fresh flowers, candles, essential oils, or bath salts, and expand your self-care regimen.

DISCOVER MORE:

essential oils; mood oils; grounding scents (musk or camphor); cooling scents (rose and lemongrass); stimulating scents (cinnamon and basil); aromatherapy

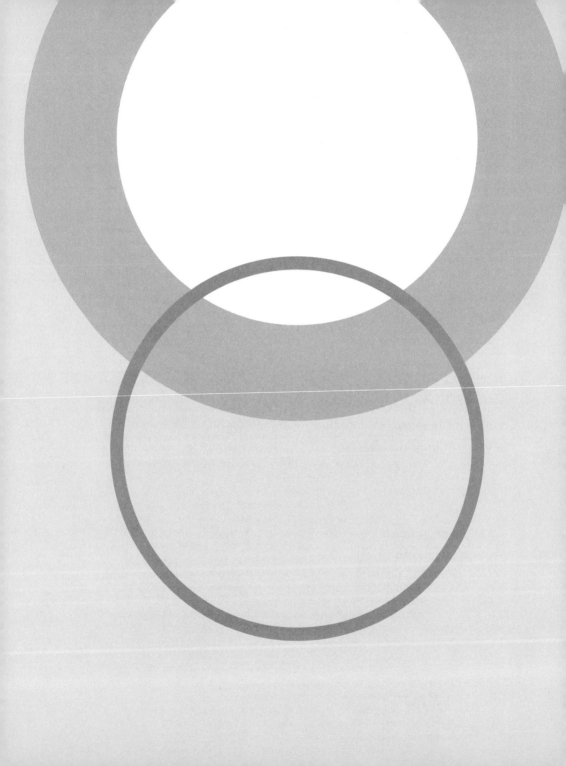

JAYNE BABINE

I am a wife, and a mother to my three-and-a-half-year-old daughter, and am re-identifying and redefining my career as a working mother, while trying to keep life in balance without losing myself and disregarding my own needs. Five years ago, my daily routine changed forever, as I stopped using body moisturizer and replaced it with a massage oil blend. I found an incredible Ayurvedic practitioner in New York City who introduced me to her doshic body oils. She advised me to use her proprietary blend of *Vata dosha* balancing massage oil between our regular monthly massage sessions. After five years of regular monthly Ayurvedic massages and integrating the body oil blends with my post-shower routine (see Tranquil Shower, page 58), I felt profound changes to my vibrational awareness, which helped me manage my demanding and stressful career in media and advertising data analytics and technology. I felt the need to seek a deeper understanding of Ayurveda in a classroom setting and to meet other like-minded, interesting people. My energetic senses have opened up, gained in strength, and led me to discover other modalities like sound healing, which I also now enjoy in regular sessions. During my work sabbatical in September 2017, I enrolled and became certified in a level-one aromatherapy program to learn about the healing properties of essential oils.

TRANQUIL SHOWER

THOUGHT BUBBLE:

"As a new mom, I want to keep life in balance without disregarding my own needs."

SIMPLE ANCIENT RITUAL:

- Pick a nourishing oil that is right for your skin type (coconut oil is generally a good choice).
- After showering, moisturize the entire body using the oil.
- Massage the body specifically in circular motions around the elbow, knee, and ankle joints.
- Massage the abdomen in the direction of the flow of indigestible matter through the colon: upward on the right abdomen, across right to left at the top of the abdomen, and then downward on the left abdomen.

MASTERY QUOTE:

"Youth fades; love droops; the leaves of friendship fall; a mother's secret hope outlives them all."
—Oliver Wendell Holmes

MODERN TAKE:

Ayurveda generally advises that a massage stroke occur eight to ten times per focus area. However, the quality of the pressure applied and the attention given is equally important. The soft and moist properties of water flowing over the body can affect vibrational energy, so a tranquil shower, along with the benefits of self-massage and aroma, will recharge you.

DISCOVER MORE:

essential oils; aromatherapy; sound healing; water therapy

ZONING

CLEARING CLUTTERED SPACE

WE ARE INTERWOVEN networks of energy, and steady energy flow is essential to our well-being. This flow also affects those we spend time with every day. An unsteady flow creates unwanted stress, such as anxiety, lethargy, despondency, anger, and burn-out. Ancient practitioners cleared these stressors by following the principle that energy cannot be created or destroyed. For instance, if you take on everyone else's problems and worry incessantly, layers of energy pile on and inhibit you, creating anxiety. If you are too sedentary, you will feel sluggish or lethargic. If you are antisocial, you will feel disconnected and, over time, may become despondent. If you hold inside the words that you need to express, eventually you will blow a gasket and feel anger. If you do not focus your attention and instead spread yourself too thin, you will eventually burn out.

The good news is this principle brings insight to our own energy habits. Each of these stressors can be addressed with energy management techniques. The more you understand your own energy pattern, the more you can direct or preserve your unique demands. Think about your body as a neighborhood with zoning laws, with boundaries to keep things apart that are incompatible in order to enable better collaboration. In practice, zoning is used to preserve the identity of the neighborhood. In my New York City neighborhood, zoning governs the height of apartment buildings, the allocation of parking spaces, the number of traffic lanes, and even outdoor seating on the sidewalks outside local restaurants. Otherwise, the neighborhood would not be livable. Rigorous planning accounts for a number of factors that will maintain the character and charm of the neighborhood. Exceptions can be granted if problems come up, but zoning maintains order so everyone can peacefully coexist.

Ancient energy gurus applied zoning laws by identifying seven energy centers that exist along our spine, from the base of the neck to the tailbone. Each center is labeled with a specific color and has sensorial tools to keep the center clean and flowing; all seven of these color zones work together so that your overall energy is maintained and flows steadily. Color is important here because it's both symbolic and a basic ingredient of energy management. Our daily experiences are shaped by the colors in our life—from our wardrobe and the food on our plate to the change of the seasons and the sports jerseys we wear for the team we support. They are also attached to the energy of our bodies, which constantly balance the layers of energy that circulate throughout the seven centers or color zones. These centers are intricately connected to our nervous and endocrine systems that affect metabolism, tissue function, growth, and even mood. When all that energy is flowing, you feel good, so care is required to keep these centers open and in balance.

Ancient practitioners called these seven color centers chakras, which means "spinning wheels." Chakras are arranged vertically from the base of the spine to the crown of the head; they are associated with both varying energy waves and the colors of the rainbow: red, orange, yellow, green, blue, indigo, and violet— also known as ROYGBIV (a helpful acronym for remembering the order of these colors). Of course, many of us can see red, orange, yellow, green, blue, indigo, and violet with our eyes. But guess what? There is a rainbow around our body when all of our energy centers are flowing steadily. I know it sounds weird, but when we talk about being a part of an energy grid, we mean that our body emits a rainbow that seeks to align with other rainbows in the world. If you are constantly stressed or worried, or live and work in a state of fear, the energy of your body can become frenzied and even blocked. Our body has a weather vane that is connected to a network of energy circuits that constantly informs our individual body parts on how to function in the moment. We know when we are in the zone—we feel good. But by slowing down and truly listening to the natural sounds of our body, we can ease our burdens and guide the well-being of our body and mind, as well as acknowledge the emotions that swirl around us. The following techniques will help you think about the structure of your body in a way that can help your energy flow better.

RED OR R-ZONE

THOUGHT BUBBLE:

"I am so upset. I cannot believe this is happening."

SIMPLE ANCIENT RITUAL:

- Find a quiet space and sit comfortably.
- Close your eyes and take a few deep breaths through your nose.
- Visualize a red spinning wheel of energy around your spine near the tailbone.
- Label it your R-zone, and imagine that area lighting up with warm, bright red energy.
- Take a few minutes to notice any thoughts, feelings, or memories that pop into your mind.
- Repeat this affirmation to yourself a few times: "I am steady and grounded."
- Sit quietly for a few minutes.
- Slowly open your eyes and take another deep, cleansing breath.

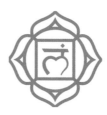

*"Everything we experience—no matter how unpleasant
—comes into our lives to teach us something."*
—Iyanla Vanzant

MODERN TAKE:

This zone helps you put fear aside and be totally present. When
the R-zone is uncluttered, you feel supported by your body; you
can draw upon this zone as an endless supply of stabilizing energy.
When this zone becomes cluttered, you feel scattered and drained.
You might shut down easily and have difficulty taking feedback.
Cleaning out the R-zone helps you feel more secure and confident
to simply be you. The several aromas that catalyze the clearing for
energy to flow include patchouli, clove, and vetiver.

DISCOVER MORE:

root chakra; color red meaning; vitality; earth; rubies; adrenal
gland; *bija mantralam*; red jasper; centered; *jin shin*

ORANGE OR O-ZONE

THOUGHT BUBBLE:

"I am so uninspired . . . listless, whatever."

SIMPLE ANCIENT RITUAL:

- Find a quiet space and sit comfortably.
- Close your eyes and take a few deep breaths through your nose.
- Visualize an orange spinning wheel of energy just below your belly button.
- Label it your O-zone, and imagine that area lighting up with warm, bright orange energy.
- Take a few minutes to notice any thoughts, feelings, or memories that pop into your mind.
- Repeat this affirmation to yourself a few times: "I feel content."
- Sit quietly for a few minutes.
- Slowly open your eyes and take another deep, cleansing breath.

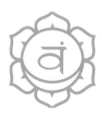

"The person who sends out positive thoughts
activates the world around him positively
and draws back to himself positive results."
—Norman Vincent Peale

MODERN TAKE:

This zone helps give you a sense of belonging and a sense of humor. It can also help you use your emotions positively, rather than being a victim to them. When the O-zone becomes cluttered, you are irritable, uninspired, and find yourself operating on autopilot. Cleaning out the O-zone ensures that you can express yourself without holding back, while still feeling compassionate. Among several aromas that catalyze the clearing for energy to flow are geranium, sandalwood, and ylang-ylang.

DISCOVER MORE:

sacral chakra; *bija mantra vum*; aventurine; color orange meaning; lotus flower; emotions; moonstone; meditation; *jin shin*

YELLOW OR Y-ZONE

THOUGHT BUBBLE:

"I do not like who I am right now."

SIMPLE ANCIENT RITUAL:
- Find a quiet space and sit comfortably.
- Close your eyes and take a few deep breaths through your nose.
- Visualize a yellow spinning wheel of energy between your chest and naval.
- Label it your Y-zone, and imagine that area lighting up with warm, bright yellow energy.
- Take a few minutes to notice any thoughts, feelings, or memories that pop into your mind.
- Repeat this affirmation to yourself a few times: "I am a force of light."
- Sit quietly for a few minutes.
- Slowly open your eyes and take another deep, cleansing breath.

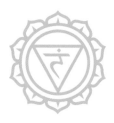

*"I must be willing to give up what I am
in order to become what I will be."*
—Albert Einstein

MODERN TAKE:

This ritual is a good way to start the day, as it puts you in a mind-set to tackle the day's challenges with optimism and self-assurance. This zone is a source of decisive confidence that helps you address problems more easily. When the Y-zone becomes cluttered, you feel angry and experience mental blocks. Cleaning out the Y-zone motivates you to achieve goals with bubbly self-confidence. Among several aromas that catalyze the clearing for energy to flow are lavender, rosemary, peppermint, and chamomile.

DISCOVER MORE:

solar plexus chakra; color yellow meaning; spleen; fire; citrine; *manipura*; *bija mantra ram*; bow pose

GREEN OR G-ZONE

THOUGHT BUBBLE:

"I want to be more optimistic about the future."

SIMPLE ANCIENT RITUAL:

- Find a quiet space and sit comfortably.
- Close your eyes and take a few deep breaths through your nose.
- Visualize a green spinning wheel of energy flowing around your heart.
- Label it your G-zone, and imagine that area lighting up with warm, bright green energy.
- Take a few minutes to notice any thoughts, feelings, or memories that pop into your mind.
- Say this affirmation to yourself a few times: "I love me better than anyone else."
- Sit quietly for a few minutes and feel the sense of calm.
- Slowly open your eyes and take another deep, cleansing breath.

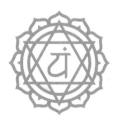

*"The future belongs to those who believe in
the beauty of their dreams."*
—Eleanor Roosevelt

MODERN TAKE:

This zone is all about your love for others as well as yourself, which is vital in order to feel a sense of harmony. It is a source of both sympathy and empathy for others. When the G-zone becomes cluttered, you might feel down and not want to socialize with people. Cleaning out the G-zone enables harmony and love and connection with others. The several aromas that catalyze the clearing for energy to flow include jasmine and marjoram.

DISCOVER MORE:

heart chakra; color green meaning; thymus gland; rose quartz; *bija mantra yam*; *anahata*; *balasana*; seed mantra

BLUE OR B-ZONE

THOUGHT BUBBLE:

"I am constantly apologizing! But for what?"

SIMPLE ANCIENT RITUAL:

- Find a quiet space and sit comfortably.
- Close your eyes and take a few deep breaths through your nose.
- Visualize a blue spinning wheel of energy around your throat.
- Label it your B-zone, and imagine that area lighting up with warm, bright blue energy.
- Take a few minutes to notice any thoughts, feelings, or memories that pop into your mind.
- Repeat this affirmation to yourself a few times: "I say what I mean, and I mean what I say."
- Sit quietly for a few minutes and feel the sense of calm.
- Slowly open your eyes and take another deep, cleansing breath.

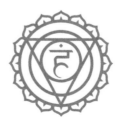

*"It took me quite a long time to develop a voice,
and now that I have it, I am not going to be silent."*
—Madeleine K. Albright

MODERN TAKE:

This zone deals with expression and helpful communication. It is a source of creativity and the flow of ideas and thoughts. When the B-zone becomes cluttered, your voice probably sounds shaky; you apologize constantly, or feel rejected and struggle to express yourself. Cleaning out the B-zone enables your voice to speak its truth with confidence and not be misunderstood by others. Among several aromas that catalyze the clearing for energy to flow are rosemary, grapefruit, sage, and frankincense.

DISCOVER MORE:

color blue meaning; throat chakra; angelite; *bija mantra ham;* cat-cow stretch; *shakini;* thyroid; *vishuddha*

INDIGO OR I-ZONE

THOUGHT BUBBLE:

"I just need to trust my gut and make a decision."

SIMPLE ANCIENT RITUAL:

- Find a quiet space and sit comfortably.
- Close your eyes and take a few deep breaths through your nose.
- Visualize a violet spinning wheel of energy between your eyebrows.
- Label it your I-zone, and imagine that area lighting up with dark bluish energy.
- Take a few minutes to notice any thoughts, feelings, or memories that pop into your mind.
- Repeat this affirmation to yourself a few times: "I see clearly."
- Sit quietly for a few minutes and feel the sense of calm.
- Slowly open your eyes and take another deep, cleansing breath.

"There is deep wisdom within our very flesh,
if we can only come to our senses and feel it."
—Elizabeth A. Behnke

MODERN TAKE:

This zone correlates with your intuition and trusting your gut. It is a source of insight and keeping mentally fit. When the I-zone becomes cluttered, you may overthink everything and feel paralyzed in making decisions. Cleaning out the I-zone can ease mental blocks and expand capacity and resourcefulness to deal with challenges and unforeseen consequences. Among several aromas that catalyze the clearing for energy to flow are orange, mint, and jasmine.

DISCOVER MORE:

color indigo meaning; ESP/intuition; mint; jasmine; *ajna* chakra; third eye; *bija mantra om;* lapis

VIOLET OR V-ZONE

THOUGHT BUBBLE:

"I feel disconnected from everything happening in my life."

SIMPLE ANCIENT RITUAL:

- Find a quiet space and sit comfortably.
- Close your eyes and take a few deep breaths through your nose.
- Visualize a violet spinning wheel of energy as a crown on your head.
- Label it your V-zone, and imagine that area lighting up with violet energy.
- Take a few minutes to notice any thoughts, feelings, or memories that pop into your mind.
- Repeat this affirmation to yourself a few times: "I now understand."
- Sit quietly for a few minutes and feel the sense of calm.
- Slowly open your eyes and take another deep cleansing breath.

"The best thing you could do is master the chaos in you.
You are not thrown into the fire; you are the fire."
—Mama Indigo

MODERN TAKE:

This zone is about wisdom and extraordinary, selfless leadership. It is a source of understanding and open-mindedness. When the V-zone becomes cluttered, you may feel chronic exhaustion, a lack of purpose, and disconnected from nature. Cleaning out the V-zone can shift your outlook and help you feel more joy by noticing your own charm in the beauty that surrounds you. The world is truly magical. The several aromas that catalyze the clearing for energy to flow include lotus, frankincense, and angelica.

DISCOVER MORE:

crown chakra; color violet meaning; higher self; empathy; clear quartz; silence; sandalwood; amethyst

QUIET ZONE

THOUGHT BUBBLE:

"I feel frazzled and need time to think."

SIMPLE ANCIENT RITUAL:

- Find a quiet space and sit comfortably.
- Close your eyes and take a few deep breaths through your nose.
- Scan all of your ROYGBIV zones one by one.
- Take a few minutes to notice any particular zone that stands out more than others.
- Give yourself a minute to identify any emotions or thoughts that pop up.
- Say the zone or zones' affirmation(s) to yourself.
- Sit quietly for a few minutes and feel the flow between the zones.
- Slowly open your eyes and take another deep, cleansing breath.

MASTERY QUOTE:

"Be silent. That heart speaks without tongue or lips."
—Rumi

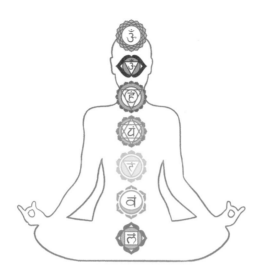

MODERN TAKE:

When life becomes noisy and stressful, simply taking the time to be quiet can soothe our nerves. Taking a few moments to stop and pause in silence also allows us to see things that we may miss when we are in a hurry. Rituals such as this one—as well as prayer, meditation, and yoga—provide a structured framework for achieving this soothing and can help us to reconnect with our selves.

DISCOVER MORE:

silence; monasteries; zazen; silent retreats; mindfulness; chakra mudras; breathing exercises

GOOD VIBE POEM

THOUGHT BUBBLE:

"I need to shake myself out of this rut!"

SIMPLE ANCIENT RITUAL:

The following are a series of sounds that, when said in order, make up what I call the "Good Vibe Poem." When you make each sound, hold the vibration for three to five seconds before moving on to the next sound.

- Say OH, as in buffalo (for the red zone).
- Say OO, as in tattoo (for the orange zone).
- Say AH, as in loofah (for the yellow zone).
- Say AY, as in hurray (for the green zone).
- Say EE, as in creek (for the blue zone).
- Say MMMM (for the indigo zone).
- Say ING, as in texting (for the violet zone).

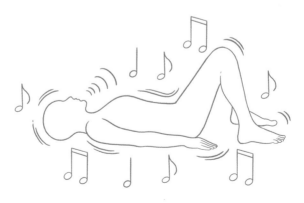

"You are precisely as big as what you love and precisely as small as what you allow to annoy you."
—Robert Anton Wilson

MODERN TAKE:

Using sound vibration to balance energy is an ancient practice that is utilized more than we may realize—with musical notes from handmade instruments, drumming, singing alone or in groups, poetry slams, and even rants that are intended to have a positive outcome. Blocked energy centers respond to the repetition of a varying frequency of sounds created by words corresponding to their respective zones, and ancient gurus believed our organ function improved when exposed to different sounds. I went through a phase when I sang loudly in the shower, making up different melodies for expressing the "Good Vibe Poem." It felt good, and it reminded me of when I was a kid and would pretend to be at the piano on a big stage belting out made-up songs. Use these sounds any way you like to help your energy flow better.

DISCOVER MORE:

chanting; poetry slam; *nada* yoga; *raga chikitsa*; throat singing

RE-ZONE

THOUGHT BUBBLE:

"There is so much clutter, it is weighing me down."

SIMPLE ANCIENT RITUAL:

- Pick a space—a cabinet, a corner, a closet—that overwhelms you with its clutter.
- Grab a garbage bag or large disposal container and set a timer for 15 minutes.
- Toss out any item that is broken or hasn't been used in years.
- Set aside any unbroken, usable item that does not serve you or feels emotionally heavy, and either recycle or donate it.
- Repeat once every week (one hour per month equals massive decluttering).

MASTERY QUOTE:

"Clutter is not just physical stuff; it's old ideas,
toxic relationships, and bad habits."
—*Eleanor Brown*

MODERN TAKE:

Intentionally managing the flow of energy throughout a physical space was derived from an ancient practice called feng shui, which originated in China. The purpose of feng shui is to create harmony with people and the "invisible forces" that enable us to coexist as we work and live. Today many people apply the principles of feng shui in modern and symbolic ways, which include decluttering one's space. When stuff piles up, it can be overwhelming, but clearing counters, cabinets, bookshelves, closets, junk drawers, or desktops in fifteen-minute sprints is enough to jump-start an energy makeover. The next time you're bored at home or have some time to spare, try cleaning out a closet or a drawer, and notice how the energy of the space changes for the better.

DISCOVER MORE:

declutter; feng shui; the *Zangshu*; yin and yang theory; *bagua*; *konmari*; *samhain* cleaning; *osouji*

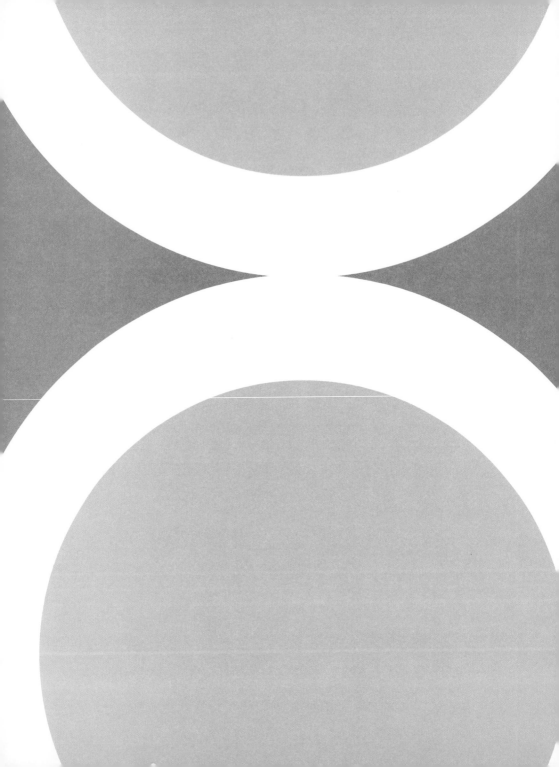

JULIA WEEKES

I was a sickly, anxious child who grew into a sickly, anxious adult. Every few years, I was diagnosed with a new autoimmune condition. In between the diagnoses, my ever-growing cadre of doctors would scratch their heads at my mysterious symptoms, offering pills to suppress them. A rheumatologist diagnosed me with systemic lupus erythematosus. All the pills and tests and doctors didn't make me healthier. I grew sicker and more anxious. I had two little boys who needed me. I knew I had to stop being a victim of my body and, instead, learn to listen to what it was telling me. It told me it was sad, angry, and scared.

It's been fifteen years since the diagnosis. For ten years, I committed my time to listening to my body and practicing kind and healing acts (see Judge-Free Zone, page 88). These have included energy work, sound meditation, guided imagery, manadala drawing, qigong, and forest bathing. I am now healthy, happy, and strong. I don't practice the same way these days. All of that good work is still in me, but now I sing and dance, listen, laugh a lot, talk to animals and trees, and notice wonderful things. This is my practice.

JUDGE-FREE ZONE

THOUGHT BUBBLE:

"I am responsible for the energy I put out in the world and for the energy I choose to take in."

SIMPLE ANCIENT RITUAL:

- Listen without judgment and notice if judgment pops in while you are listening.
- As you listen, focus on each word and the message being delivered.
- Ask the speaker if they are ready to hear your response.
- Repeat back the main message that you heard and ask if it was accurate.
- Respond with words that are easily accepted and convey understanding.
- Suspend your own beliefs.

MASTERY QUOTE:

"Every time you smile at someone, it is an action of love, a gift to that person, a beautiful thing."
—*Mother Teresa*

MODERN TAKE:

If I am responsible for the energy I put out into the world, then I need to pay close attention to my own gestures, body language, and words as I engage in conversation. As you practice this ritual—suspending belief—focus on how well you listen and the tone and words that shape the reply. This ensures that the energy is clean versus misjudging what other people say or mean. Choose to respond with words that can be more easily heard while always working toward greater empathy. Relationships with loved ones and coworkers will be richer, warmer, and more fulfilling. And when there are no words, just smile and play a positive part in maintaining the positive energy.

DISCOVER MORE:

active listening; blame; serendipity; karma; *upekkha*; chamomile; essential oils

SHIFTING

CHANGING THINGS UP

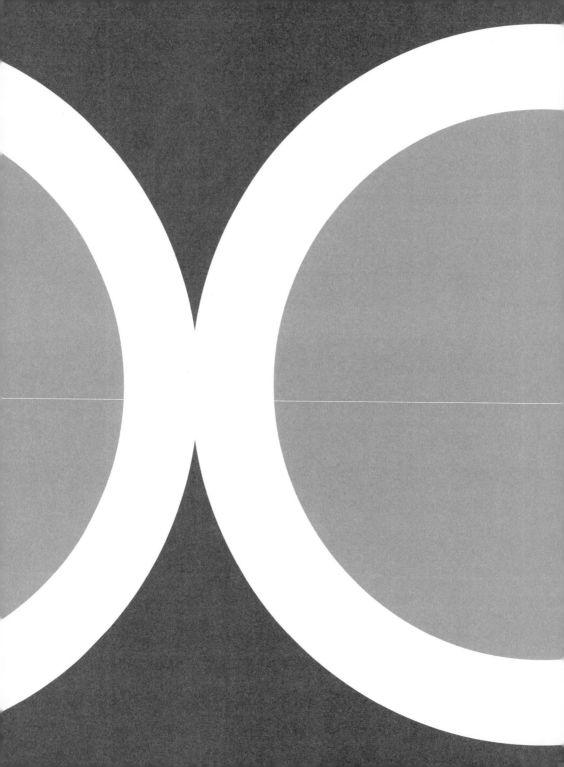

DARIA KALININA

I am a thirty-three-year-old holistic life enthusiast. About five years ago, I experienced a physical and mental break-down. I was suffering from excruciating menstrual pain, rapid weight gain, adult acne, mood swings, insomnia followed by severe lethargy—the list goes on. It felt as if an alien had taken over my body and was now in control. I certainly did not feel like me. After a year of many trips to sterile doctors' offices and receiving false diagnoses, I not only did not have any relief from my symptoms, I had no helpful solutions. I decided to take my health into my own hands. I bought every health book I could find and started to study the systems of my body. I participated in several detoxification programs and started to feel better and more like myself again. A few months into my quest to gain my health back, I stumbled upon Ayurveda. Every word I read had a profound resonance with some of the issues I was experiencing and showed me ways to bring my body back into balance. It was so inspiring I enrolled in a certification program at Ayurveda World shortly after. After the program was over, my health had dramatically improved. I then decided to complete a 200-hour yoga teacher training at SuperSoul Farm, as well as an iridology program at New York Center for Iridology. I became my own test kitchen, trying every recipe, herb, superfood, yoga posture, and *pranayama*. After five years, I am happier and healthier than I could ever have imagined, and my own holistic healing is a testament to others who helped me uncover ways to get my health back. Now I want to share what my life was like before taking a holistic approach and ways that I shifted, as well as describe the rituals that have now become my routine and changed my outlook on life.

Shifting a little bit every day had a dramatic impact on my health over time. First off, gone are the days of sleeping past noon, waking up groggy, bloated, and still feeling tired. I used to rush out of the house having just brushed my teeth and gotten dressed, only to show up late to wherever I was heading, usually with some kind of sugary, dense granola bar in hand. My routine is so different now. It took roughly a year to incorporate all the rituals that have now become my new normal daily routine. While incorporating new rituals changed my life, the benefits were quite clear from the start. By adapting these simple changes, I noticed improvements in my own emotional intelligence and physical agility. Going with the flow has become second nature. I wake up and begin my day around 5:30 a.m., or just before sunrise (see A.M. Wake-Up Call, page 98). There is something extraordinarily magical about this time of day. I splash cool water on my face and then reach for my nifty tongue scraper (see Tongue Scraping, page 100). If my scraper is clean, I know my body is getting what it needs (see Tongue IQ, page 46).

Next, I swish a spoonful of organic coconut oil around in my mouth (see Oil Pulling, page 102). It took a while to get used to this technique, but the benefits of cleaner breath and less infection is worth it. Then it's time for a big glass of warm water with lemon. Even if I am traveling or am somewhere remote, I never skip this step. This drink releases toxins and helps to regulate natural bowel movements—after evacuating my bowel, I sit down to practice breathwork.

There are countless books written on the practice and benefits of *pranayama*, or breathwork (see Breath IQ, page 4). I have had the opportunity to study with incredible gurus including Dr. Vasant Lad who taught me the eight pranayama breaths during an intensive at the Ayurvedic Institute in New Mexico. This enabled me to enhance my understanding of these ancient breathing rituals and see the positive impact on my practice. If you only have ten minutes in the morning and have to make a choice between breathwork and stretching, choose breathwork every time. If I have more time, I practice stretching for about forty-five minutes. My practice changes daily, according to what my body needs and craves that day. Whether it's a yin or a yang practice, it leaves me clearheaded and feeling strong. A home practice is sacred, but I also love taking classes and being part of the yoga community. Never tried yoga? Feeling intimidated? Going with a friend or taking a community class is a great way to start. Yoga increases flexibility, relieves stress, and creates balance within the body. More and more wellness practices prescribe yoga for improving the health of the body. I conclude my physical practice with a short silent meditation. Whether it's just five minutes of silence or an intentional ten minutes of So-Hum meditation (see Clean Slate, page 10), this practice helps clear my mind, so that the rest of the day I can process information better, stay calmer, and make better decisions. Then it is time for a cleansing shower.

Abhyanga is a form of Ayurvedic medicine that involves massaging the body with *dosha*-specific infused oils (see Self-Massage, page 52). Depending on the time of year and my physical state, I will choose from sesame, sunflower, or coconut oil, or an herbal infusion. I warm the oil, applying it to my body in a circular motion, starting at the inner thigh and working my way down the legs with upward motions. Once the lower body is complete, I work on the wrists, working my way up the arms, around the breast, then in a U-shape following the large intestine. This is a great time to give thanks for my physical body and show it love and care. At first, this felt uncomfortable, but now I relish every moment in a mood of gratitude for this vehicle that works so hard 24/7—never resting, constantly healing, and working toward my benefit. The benefits include but are not limited to bringing moisture to the skin, soothing *Vata* imbalance, cleansing *ama* through the skin, increasing stamina throughout the day, and much more. At this point, the sun has risen, and my belly is growling; it's breakfast time. According to Ayurveda, lunch is the biggest meal of the day. I find this hard to do on certain days, so I make breakfast my biggest meal of the day, with lunch the second biggest. My favorite breakfast is *khichdi* topped with a dollop of ghee (see Preparing a Pot of *Khichdi* recipe on page 110). It is a one-pot dish that is easy and quick and is excellent for detoxification. It has become a staple meal, and I mix it up by adding fresh vegetables, spices, and fresh herbs that are available.

My morning routine is grounding and sets the mood for the rest of the day. I make better decisions, am kinder to coworkers and family, and feel a sense of ease and vitality like never before. I am eternally grateful to my teachers for passing down this ancient wisdom. I hope to keep these practices alive for many years to come and share them with others. My evening routine has also changed and you will learn more about it in my spotlight on page 121.

A.M. WAKE-UP CALL

THOUGHT BUBBLE:

"I feel so rushed in the morning."

SIMPLE ANCIENT RITUAL:

- Set your alarm for five minutes before sunrise.
- When you wake up, resist going back to sleep.
- Lie in bed and imagine the sun rising outside your door to greet you.
- Hear the sun give you the light you need to flow throughout your day.
- Give your mind the space to allow your thoughts to flow.
- Listen to yourself and accept what you are thinking.
- Identify one task you will accomplish today and give yourself a pep talk.
- Remind yourself of the gift of getting up early so you do not feel as rushed or stressed.

MASTERY QUOTE:

"Early to bed and early to rise makes a man healthy, wealthy, and wise."
—*Proverb*

MODERN TAKE:

Cycles are a natural part of life, and Ayurveda teaches the importance of living in tune with nature. This includes the daily sleep-wake cycle that ancient gurus believed should mirror the rising and setting of the sun. Constantly being "on" and disconnected from nature can take its toll on us, and especially on the quality of our sleep. Seasonal cycles require time for adapting to the changes in weather as well as the lengths of the day. While modern life has made us more dependent on man-made things, waking up with the sun can give you a positive, natural start to the day.

DISCOVER MORE:

circadian rhythm; melatonin; seasonal affective disorder; light therapy; vitamin D

TONGUE SCRAPING

THOUGHT BUBBLE:

"My breath smells disgusting in the morning."

SIMPLE ANCIENT RITUAL:
- Stick out your tongue and notice its appearance.
- Pick your scraper of choice; you can likely use the back of the toothbrush, but you can also purchase a dedicated tongue-scraper if you'd prefer.
- Gently scrape your tongue, using a downward motion.
- Repeat five times.
- Rinse the scraper while noticing the color and thickness of the residue.

MASTERY QUOTE:

"A man too busy to take care of his health is like a mechanic too busy to take care of his tools."
—*Spanish proverb*

MODERN TAKE:

Paying attention to oral care goes beyond brushing and flossing the teeth. Scraping the tongue every morning to remove any residue can improve your taste and breath, and maintain healthier saliva.

DISCOVER MORE:

ama; oral hygiene; bad breath; *agni*; Ayurveda tongue map

OIL PULLING

THOUGHT BUBBLE:

"I've brushed my teeth, but is the inside of my mouth really clean?"

SIMPLE ANCIENT RITUAL:

- Place a small amount of coconut oil on a spoon.
- Put the spoon in your mouth, and if it is not liquid yet, let it melt.
- Swish the oil around inside your mouth, but do not swallow it.
- Direct the oil around the teeth and gums.
- Swish in your mouth for 2-3 minutes.
- Spit it out into the trash can (not into the sink, as it will clog the drain).

MASTERY QUOTE:

"They sure are handy when you smile,
so keep your teeth around a while."
—Dr. Seuss

MODERN TAKE:

Ancient practitioners used fennel and *triphala* to cleanse the sensitive tissues of the mouth, but today many people use coconut oil instead, so keep a jar on hand for everyday use. It took a while for me to grow accustomed to this technique, as it feels odd to have oil in your mouth. But I chose to focus on its benefits, such as pulling out toxins that may be on your tongue, removing film that may be covering the taste buds, and helping get rid of plaque and harmful bacteria.

DISCOVER MORE:

oil pulling; daily swish; oral hygiene; *kavala*; coconut oil

TRANSITIONING

WELCOMING HOPEFUL SERENDIPITY

TRANSITIONS SIGNAL CHANGE. Even if we do not believe we are ready for drastic change, it is important to identify ways to transition for significant change in your life. One of the best examples I can remember is when my children began preschool. During the first week, I didn't leave them at the front door and pick them up at the end of the day. The first day consisted of me waiting outside the preschool for a couple of hours after dropping them off in the event they needed me and then taking them home. The second day was a little bit longer, and each consecutive day was longer than that, until my children had enough confidence in the fact that this was now a new routine in their daily lives. Developing new daily constructs, as well as personal relationships to support the intention, seems to fall off our radars when we dive into new routines and expect them to stick right away. The same applies for our body and mind needing space for transitions. If you believe there are stages to acquiring new habits, then you know that, at the end of everything, there is some kind of immediate benefit or reward. Some goals take longer than others, and it is essential to break goals down into smaller steps so that each in their own right signals being on a clear path toward the goal.

Breakfast is the first meal of the day, and its name ("break fast") signals the end of the fasting period of the prior night. While most experts believe it is the most important meal of the day in terms of its effect on health, there is still more to learn about breakfast and its role on holistic health. Many cultures have different beliefs about breakfast that caused me to rethink mine. For example, in India, there are more than twenty-five types of breakfasts that include hundreds of different types of foods, instead of the few standard breakfasts we often eat in the United States.

It raises the question *Why do we accept the notions surrounding breakfast that have been handed down to us, and not think more about our holistic needs that may shift from day to day?* The following rituals will explore both how and what we eat, in general (i.e., not just at breakfast), can serve our holistic needs and improve our overall well-being.

BREAK | FAST

THOUGHT BUBBLE:

"I want to wake up and feel energized for the day."

SIMPLE ANCIENT RITUAL:

- Intentionally acknowledge the new day by saying aloud, "Today is a fresh start."
- Prepare a beverage of your choosing and make a toast to the sun for bringing light to a new day.
- Mix it up on the weekend by making a tea blend prepared in a French press.
- Add loose-leaf black tea, fresh ginger, lemon, rosemary, and sage to the French press.
- Feel free to also mix any combination of tea (green, black, herbal), citrus, herb, and essence.
- Take time to enjoy the flavor of what you've brewed.

MASTERY QUOTE:

"Often when you think you're at the end of something, you're at the beginning of something else."
—Fred Rogers

MODERN TAKE:

A fresh start awaits you every morning. While breakfast may be touted as the most important meal of the day, acknowledging the transition with the mind-set of a new beginning is equally important. Creating structure for waking up and practicing new rituals to greet the day has noticeably increased my energy capacity and overall ability to manage what comes my way without emotional drama. Yes, I have moments when I deviate from this new routine, and they are generally followed by my own sense of strain as I try to handle all that needs my time and attention. But I encourage you to own the mornings and celebrate each one as a fresh start to a new beginning.

DISCOVER MORE:

san-Senke; tea ceremony; tea nook; green tea; French press

PREPARING A POT OF *KHICHDI*

THOUGHT BUBBLE:

"I don't have time to prepare wholesome meals every day."

SIMPLE ANCIENT RITUAL:

Ingredients:
- 4 tablespoons coconut oil
- 1/4 teaspoon mustard seeds
- 1/4 teaspoon cumin seeds
- 1/4 cup chopped mint leaves
- 6 curry leaves
- 1/2 cup rice (e.g., jasmine or brown), rinsed
- 1/2 cup mung beans, washed and soaked
- 3 cups water
- 1 cup grated coconut
- 1 tablespoon of tamarind (or mango pulp)
- 3/4 cup chopped coriander leaves
- 1 teaspoon chopped ginger
- 1 teaspoon minced garlic
- 1 cup chopped vegetables (e.g., baby kale or spinach)
- 1 tablespoon grated jaggery

Instructions:
1. Add coconut oil to a large pot.
2. After the pot becomes hot, add the mustard seeds, cumin seeds, mint leaves and curry leaves, and brown them for a minute to release their flavor.
3. Add rice, mung beans, and 2 of the 3 cups of water.
4. Cook the rice and beans until they are soft and mushy.

5. In a blender, add grated coconut, tamarind or mango, most of the coriander, ginger, and garlic, and blend well.
6. Add the coconut-based blended puree to the rice and beans after they are fully cooked.
7. Add remaining 1 cup of water, chopped vegetables, and jaggery.
8. Boil and simmer for 10–15 minutes on low heat until the vegetables are cooked.
9. Top the dish off with the remaining chopped coriander leaves.

Serving Size: 1 cup. Makes 6 cups.

MASTERY QUOTE:

*"One cannot think well, love well, sleep well,
if one has not dined well."*
—Virginia Woolf

MODERN TAKE:

There are many ways to prepare *khichdi*, including this easy-to-digest stew that can be a pick-me-up in the middle of the week or nourishment during a detoxification plan (see *Khichdi*, page 152). Make a large pot with extra beans and rice and set aside a portion; then add different vegetables and spices throughout a busy week for additional wholesome meals.

DISCOVER MORE:

khichdi recipes; tridoshic; mung dahl beans; complete protein; digestive health

WARM GOLDEN MILK

THOUGHT BUBBLE:

"I love a nightly ritual, but I don't want to drink alcohol."

SIMPLE ANCIENT RITUAL:

Ingredients

- 1–1 1/2 cups light coconut milk (or any type of milk)
- 1 1/2 teaspoon ground turmeric
- 1/4 teaspoon ground ginger
- 1 whole cinnamon stick (or 1/4 teaspoon ground cinnamon)
- 1 tablespoon coconut oil
- A dash of pepper (optional)
- honey or other sweetener, to taste
- ground cinnamon, for garnish

Instructions:

1. Place ingredients in a small saucepan.
2. Cook, stirring frequently, until the milk mixture is warm but not boiling.
3. Give it a taste, and add honey or sweetener to taste.
4. Sprinkle with ground cinnamon.

MASTERY QUOTE:

"The way you prepare the bed, so shall you sleep."
—Yiddish proverb

MODERN TAKE:

Winding down before bed is an important transition before we are able to get a solid night of sleep, and golden milk (also known as turmeric tea or turmeric latte) is a fabulous way to wind down before bedtime, although it can be enjoyed at any time of day. This nightcap is a 3,000-year-old recipe from India's holistic medical tradition that has been used for colds, congestion, headache, and sore throats—and this nourishing drink contains turmeric, which gives it a beautiful yellow color. Curcumin, turmeric's best-known compound, has medicinal properties and is commonly used to help reduce joint pain, arthritis, and inflammation. Golden milk has been helping people go to sleep and stay asleep for centuries. Why not add it to your evening routine?

DISCOVER MORE:

turmeric; golden milk; herbalism; tea nook; anti-inflammatory superfoods

CUMIN CORIANDER FENNEL (CCF) TEA BREAK

THOUGHT BUBBLE:
"I feel so heavy and bloated."

SIMPLE ANCIENT RITUAL:
- Combine equal parts cumin, coriander, and fennel seeds in a hot pan.
- Slightly heat until aroma is released.
- Pour water over the seeds and bring to a boil for 1–2 minutes.
- Turn off heat and allow to cool.
- Enjoy at any time of day.

MASTERY QUOTE:
"Drinking a daily cup of tea will surely starve the apothecary."
—Ancient Chinese proverb

MODERN TAKE:

Transitioning to different foods instead of having the same thing every day is an enabler for better digestion, and eating certain foods like raw broccoli, lettuce, onions, apples, pears, beans, lentils, and whole grains can cause bloating. Improving digestion goes beyond focusing on the individual sections of the digestive tract (i.e., esophagus, stomach, large intestine, small intestine, and rectum), and includes paying attention to the long lining of two thin layers made up of nerve cells that release the enzymes that break down food and keep it all moving. The combination of cumin, coriander, and fennel offers relief by reducing cramps, gas, and an overly acidic stomach.

DISCOVER MORE:

IBS; CCF; link between bowel and anxiety; herbalism; gut-brain connection

SILENCE IS GOLDEN

THOUGHT BUBBLE:

"I can barely function, and I just want to crawl into bed."

SIMPLE ANCIENT RITUAL:

- Over a 24-hour period, give your liver a rest by talking less and eating less food.
- Stop eating after the sun sets, and do not eat again until after the sun rises.
- Avoid sugar and alcohol to turn fat production in the liver off.
- Over a one- or two-day period, eat more complete protein, celery, carrots, and cruciferous vegetables.

MASTERY QUOTE:

"The only person you are destined to become is the person you decide to be."
—Ralph Waldo Emerson

MODERN TAKE:

The liver has an amazing ability to heal itself, and ancient gurus believe that silence is a part of that healing. Observing a moment of silence is fairly common to honor a tragic event or passing of a loved one; however, we often want to avoid silence during conversations. Now silent retreats are becoming more popular as we understand how noisy environments can take their toll on us. Silence can be deafening, too, and having a conversation with your mind is in its own right its own experience. Know it all matters and can improve with a transition plan, though. If you speak less, say more; if you never stop talking long enough to allow others to engage, then gradually tone yourself down. Pay attention to how much you contribute to the noise and the silence.

DISCOVER MORE:

liver function; fatty liver; *manipura*; intermittent fasting; meditation; Vipassana

PRACTICING

ESTABLISHING NEW ROUTINES

DARIA KALININA

It is challenging to stay up late when your everyday routine requires waking up early. Establishing structure, such as targeting a specific time to wake up and go to sleep, enables your natural body clock to sync up with its natural circadian rhythm. I am very aware of the rising and setting of the sun to nudge me to wake up or slow down. My daily work schedule changes, so I am intentional about maintaining a consistent evening routine. It requires discipline, given the opportunities to go out to join friends and family for occasional fun and celebration, but overall maintaining that consistency is key for enabling me to stay balanced since I have less flexibility at the start of my day. Whether it's a quick rinse in the shower to get the dust and dirt off or a thirty-minute bath, I am grateful for fresh, clean water to remove any stagnant or negative energy. If I have time to soak, adding calming ingredients, such as a lavender essential oil, Epsom salts, baking soda, bentonite clay, apple cider vinegar, ginger, hydrogen peroxide, or even sea salt can enhance my experience. I highly recommend you build your own pantry of go-to calming elixirs to enhance your routine. After a hot soak or a shower, my typical evening includes gentle stretching, sipping on golden milk, and adding an item to my gratitude list, as well as sending good thoughts and prayers to my family and friends. On a day when I cannot wind down, I may crank up the music and have a private dance party!

CATERPILLAR

THOUGHT BUBBLE:

"I need to do something physical to help me wind down at night."

SIMPLE ANCIENT RITUAL:

- From a seated position, extend your legs out in front of you.
- Begin to walk your hands forward on your body until you reach a sign of tension.
- Round the spine forward and relax your legs.
- Breathe with a focus on the back of your body.
- Hold for 25 breaths.

MASTERY QUOTE:

"The body benefits from movement, and the mind benefits from stillness."
—Sakyong Mipham

MODERN TAKE:

This stretch suggestion is based on yin yoga and is both very relaxing and meditative, though it's not exactly restorative, because there is much going on inside the body while practicing. Yin postures are typically held for 3–10 minutes each. This length of time for holding each posture allows the inner lining of the muscle to release. This practice also aids in flexibility, relaxation, and detoxification.

DISCOVER MORE:

yin yoga; stretching; *Utthan Pristhasana*; *Ananda Balasana*; *Viparita Karani*

GRATITUDE JOURNAL

THOUGHT BUBBLE:
"Nothing went my way today!"

SIMPLE ANCIENT RITUAL:
- Keep a journal or a sheet of paper and pen handy (or use the journal pages in the back of this book) before you go to sleep.
- Write down one thing you are grateful for.
- Continue for ten nights, adding one item to the list every night.
- Once the list includes ten items, reread the list every day for another ten days.
- Observe and reflect on your daily interactions with life, noticing how you begin to see situations differently.

MASTERY QUOTE:
*"Gratitude is a powerful catalyst for happiness.
It's the spark that lights a fire of joy in your soul."*
—Amy Collette

MODERN TAKE:

A dear colleague of mine kept a gratitude journal on a dated daily calendar. Imagine having had a calendar starting in 2001, and every day, year after year, you jotted down just one thing that made you smile. He also happened to be a songwriter, and it offered up inspiration in the midst of managing a challenging leadership position in the corporate world. Gratitude has a ripple effect, no matter how it shows up. There is nothing too great or too small for acknowledgment and appreciation. So I acknowledge the existence of my ten fingers and ten toes, clean water that comes out of a faucet or shower, a beautiful song, electricity, a handwritten note from a dear friend, a surprise windfall for paying a bill, and the accessibility of nourishing food.

DISCOVER MORE:

science of gratitude; gratitude journal; positive psychology; *Anjali Mudra*; *dhanya vad*; gratitude letters

PRAYER CHAIN

THOUGHT BUBBLE:

"My friend is in serious trouble and needs support."

SIMPLE ANCIENT RITUAL:
- Put someone or a group of people into your thoughts.
- Imagine the help they may need coming to their front door.
- Ask that they can open the door and receive the gift of help.
- Ask that others join you in supporting them with thoughts and prayers.
- Remind yourself of the wisdom of not trying to fix the problem for them.

MASTERY QUOTE:

"Heaven is full of answers to prayer for which no one bothered to ask."
—Billy Graham

MODERN TAKE:

Ask for help. A prayer is a solemn request for help or an expression of thanks, usually addressed to a god or an object of worship. Prayer may be polarizing, based on your religious beliefs, but the intent is an earnest request in order to mobilize support. I grew up in an environment where my parents received prayer requests and placed them on a weekly bulletin to engage support from our church community. This is very common to some groups, yet foreign to others. We all know people who need support and we cannot always be physically present when needed, but we can put their needs in our hearts. When praying for others, we are a conduit of positive energy and open to receiving blessings, too. If you struggle with the idea of prayer, know that it doesn't have to be addressed to anyone or anything in particular. Simply have someone or a group of people in mind, and send them positive and healthy energy.

DISCOVER MORE:

prayer; the Secret; Law of Attraction; creative visualization; manifestation habits

PRIVATE DANCE PARTY

THOUGHT BUBBLE:

"My body wants to dance, but I don't feel like getting dressed and going out with friends."

SIMPLE ANCIENT RITUAL:

- Make a three- to five-song private party playlist that lifts your spirits.
- Crank up the volume or put on your headphones, and take in the music.
- Move your body to the beat of the music.
- Keep going until you feel better!

MASTERY QUOTE:

"Dance is the hidden language of the soul."
—Martha Graham

MODERN TAKE:

A body moving to a beat of its own drum is a beautiful thing! And moving your body to music will become a saving grace once you try it. Whether you are happy or sad, having the best day ever, or the worst, movement can bring you balance. I highly recommend blasting your favorite song and moving to the groove anytime you feel the need. Dancing will work up a sweat, release unwanted emotions and energy, and put you in the present moment. It's something so natural, but we too often forget to do it. Don't feel silly, and even if you do, go with it, be even sillier, feel the inner child having a blast.

DISCOVER MORE:

movement; dance; ecstatic dance; trance dance; holistic dance; Biodanza

NATURE WALK

THOUGHT BUBBLE:

"I rarely get to play on the grass or take a walk in the woods."

SIMPLE ANCIENT RITUAL:

- Identify where and when you can take 20 minutes to get outside and breathe fresh air.
- Notice the sounds of nature around you.
- Practice deep breathing and experience gratitude for the time to walk.
- Bring nature into your work environment, such as having plants at your workspace.
- Plan a future trip to a national park and spend the day exploring.

MASTERY QUOTE:

"The clearest way into the Universe is through a forest wilderness."
—John Muir

MODERN TAKE:

When the weather permits, take a walk outside in nature. Spend at least thirty minutes in a forest or in a dense collection of trees. Certain trees have been known to possess healing and anti-cancer properties. Trees, of course, also produce oxygen, and who doesn't need more of that? Forest bathing, also known as ecotherapy, has become a technique in nature healing and is a part of treatments that have the intention of improving mental and physical health. Besides, trees have been around for more than 300 million years! Who needs more proof that they're onto something good?

DISCOVER MORE:

national parks; nature hikes; flaneuring; walkabout; walking meditation; psychogeography

OWNING

NOTICING WHAT FLOWS

THE RELENTLESS PACE of life makes it easy to slip into unhealthy patterns that limit our energy flow states. We eat on the go and make expedient choices that create ease in the moment but cause problems later. We fill our homes with wireless technology to simplify tasks without hesitation and not understanding the potential impact. Thankfully, our bodies send us signals that prompt change. The key is to learn to pay attention to these subtle cues that tell us our systems are not operating at optimal levels. This is true for both our bodies and our homes—our sacred personal spaces.

Let's start with the body. The phrase "You are what you eat" evolved from the ancient belief that what we digest becomes our strength and what we cannot digest becomes our weakness. Weakness not only shows up as physical symptoms (e.g., gas, bloating) but also as emotional symptoms, including irritation, fatigue, and sometimes fiery anger. But all of this discomfort can be reduced with an intentional practice of silence, fasting, cleansing, and rejuvenation.

The capacity and ability to digest is underappreciated, given the constant adjustments and fine-tuning needed for both the shifting conditions of the body (e.g., being ill or well), in addition to adapting to what types of food we eat (e.g., hot, cold, spicy, oily, soft, or hard). Imagine if you eat cold cereal and drink an icy drink for every meal, the stomach works harder to adequately break down what you ingest into the right consistency and move it at an optimal pace through the more than twenty feet of plumbing that is our digestive system. The speed and total transit time is important given the body requires time in the right places to extract the good stuff, like vitamins, distribute some of what is extracted to convert it into energy, and then eliminate the remaining waste. Otherwise, toxins can build up, resulting in what I call "sick" poop—sometimes sticky, loose, mucousy white, or foul-smelling waste products of incomplete digestion. Your digestive waste is a good indicator for what your body needs more or less of every day. Incorporating a variety of hot and cold nutrient-dense foods and drinks into a few rejuvenation rituals helps steady the flow of energy and revitalize digestive function.

There are many rituals that can be incorporated on a daily, weekly, seasonal, or even annual basis to restore balance to the body, mind, and emotions, including occasionally eliminating added sugar, alcohol, or stimulants such as coffee in order to improve the power of your digestion. You may also find that short- and long-term fasting will make a notable difference in your mental clarity and increased energy, especially if you commit to one between the change of the seasons. If this is new to you, start with a half-day fast and notice how it makes you feel. My first three-day liver cleanse had surprising lasting benefits, including lifting the brain fog I didn't even know I had.

The physical spaces we inhabit also need cleansing from time to time. Technology, for instance, powers our daily lives through electromagnetic fields (EMFs), but most people are unaware of the different types of EMFs, and the distinction is important. There are natural EMFs, which are emitted from sources like the sun, thunderstorm activity, and currents circulating in the core of the earth. And then there are other, more concerning EMFs that are emitted from man-made sources like Wi-Fi. Today, EMFs support an ever-expanding network of appliances, cell phones, and wireless routers that fill the spaces in our homes. In other words, we operate and sleep within an amplified grid of energy that is invisible to the eye and yet ever present.

This isn't natural, and we're beginning to realize another reason for being "on" 24/7 is not good for us either. In 2011, the International Agency for Research on Cancer labeled EMFs as "possibly carcinogenic to humans," and smartphones have been linked to everything from insomnia to mental fog to a lack of empathy. Moreover, most of us are exposed to the blue light emitted from the screens of our devices up until we go to bed. This light suppresses melatonin in the body, making us more alert when our system should naturally be shutting down to sleep. Ultimately, our digital habits have gradually overtaken our lives, and we're paying the price.

The good news is that there are a number of ways you can find your flow again, as well as begin to detox from your digital devices for the betterment of your health and well-being. Check out the following rituals that are inspired by ancient living to find your starting point.

MARYANNE O'BRIEN

I believe that life is a creative process fueled by our willingness to experiment, adapt, evolve, and transform. If someone had told me at the age of twenty that this would be my perspective at the age of fifty, I would have dismissed the notion mid-sentence. I was wired for command and control, not experiment and change.

Thankfully, my curious nature enabled me to stay open to new (and ancient) ideas. I started experimenting with practices that went against the grain of hot trends and society's norms. I studied energy healing, reduced EMF (see EMF Detox, page 138) and Wi-Fi exposure (much to my kid's displeasure), embraced detox programs, and treated food as medicine.

Every transformative experience started as I made one small change, followed by another. At first, it took intentional practice. Over time, it became a way of being. The results? I am healthy, happy, and experiencing the benefits of being consciously connected to the systems that support life on every level.

EMF DETOX

THOUGHT BUBBLE:

"I can't fall asleep. Then when I do, I wake up throughout the night."

SIMPLE ANCIENT RITUAL:
- Decrease man-made EMFs that could possibly disturb sleep.
- Make your bedroom a tech-free zone, including keeping the router out of your bedroom.
- Turn off your Wi-Fi at night to reduce unnecessary exposure and distraction.
- Avoid electronic screens for 45 minutes before sleep.
- If your phone is your alarm, put it on airplane mode.
- Keep your phone ten feet away from your body while you sleep.
- Periodically fast from all electronics, and always eliminate technology at meal time.

MASTERY QUOTE:
"Rest and be thankful."
—William Wadsworth

MODERN TAKE:

Create conscious breaks during which you are completely tech-free. Emerging studies have linked EMFs to sleep disturbances as more homes use wireless technology that is on 24/7, so try experimenting by detoxing your sleep environment, and pay attention to how the quality of your sleep improves.

DISCOVER MORE:

EMF nutrition; anti-radiation diet; faraday pouches; tourmaline shielding

SUNSET FAST

THOUGHT BUBBLE:

"I think it is time to rethink my daily routine."

SIMPLE ANCIENT RITUAL:

- Take note of the time that the sun will rise and set the next day.
- Plan out a schedule of light meals to be eaten between dawn and sunset.
- Do not eat solid food after the sun sets.
- Sip on an herbal tea during the evening.
- Go to bed around 10:00 p.m. or when ready.
- Rise at sunrise.

MASTERY QUOTE:

"Whenever you find yourself on the side of the majority, it's time to pause and reflect."
—Mark Twain

MODERN TAKE:

If we are working long hours, we often eat around the clock. This is hard on the vital organs that have to process it. Ayurveda emphasizes routine for eating and sleep as a way to combat the stressors on our daily lives. Creating consistency for when we eat has a positive effect on our overall health and well-being. Celebrate the body and its connection to the natural rhythms of the rising and the setting of the sun. Notice your overall reaction to waking up early and the times you choose to eat and record your thoughts.

DISCOVER MORE:

body natural rhythms; ketosis; religious fasting; intuitive eating; intermittent fasting

QUICK FAST

THOUGHT BUBBLE:

"I have not been taking the time to eat as well as I normally do."

SIMPLE ANCIENT RITUAL:

- Identify a half day or full day when you will not eat solid foods.
- Sip your favorite warm decaffeinated tea throughout the day to help flush out toxins.
- Do not underestimate a pause in eating for helping your body feel better.

MASTERY QUOTE:

"When you change the way you look at things, the things you look at change."
—Max Planck

MODERN TAKE:

Intermittent fasting or IF is a technique that simply means not eating during specific times. The most common form called 16:8 suggests eating only during an eight-hour window during the day and fasting for the remaining sixteen hours. A quick fast is not intended to be the entire day, but can support the inner workings of digestion, especially after a long holiday weekend of eating too much while socializing with friends and family. When this happens on occasion, I generally choose not to eat solid food on the following Monday, but more teas and smoothies. For people concerned about pre-diabetes, intermittent fasting is known to improve sensitivity to the blood glucose-lowering hormone called insulin. There are plenty of options to consider given the focus is on when to eat not what to eat.

DISCOVER MORE:

liver fast; body natural rhythms; ketosis; religious fasting; intuitive eating; intermittent fasting

ONE-DAY FAST

THOUGHT BUBBLE:
"I need to give my body a break."

SIMPLE ANCIENT RITUAL:
- Identify a full day in which you will take in only light liquids and remain quiet.
- Sip warm decaffeinated teas throughout the day to flush out toxins from your body.
- Keep on hand a journal to record the ideas or thoughts that pop in periodically.
- Identify times for breathing and stretching.

MASTERY QUOTE:
"Take care of your body. It's the only place you have to live."
—Jim Rohn

MODERN TAKE:

Just one day of silence while fasting gives the body a well-deserved break. When my holistic healing certification group participated in a silent retreat during which we ingested only basic liquids for nourishment, my body felt better and my mind became more clear and alert for the days that followed. Before these daily fasts, rejuvenation meant getting more sleep or unplugging from electronics. Now the discipline of taking a few hours or even a full day has expanded my understanding of the benefits of rejuvenation without having to leave the conveniences of home base. Writing in my journal during these experiences allowed me to compare my observations to my daily routines during the week and on the weekend. It was clear that devoting one day, or even a half of a day, to a quiet zone while consuming my favorite herbal tea blend or just hot water with lemon shifted me back into balance.

DISCOVER MORE:

liver health; fasting; detox; ketosis; body natural rhythms; religious fasting; intuitive eating; intermittent fasting

THREE-DAY
LIVER
REJUVENATION

IF YOU ARE "on" twenty-four hours per day, then so is your liver. As the largest glandular organ, located on the right side of your body near your stomach, it filters up to two liters of blood per minute, is hooked up to both the heart and the small intestine, and receives oxygen-rich blood and digested food. The liver is the center for the metabolism of all the vitamins, carbohydrates, minerals, proteins, fats, and hormones we take in and relies on your exercise, breathwork, quiet time, and solid sleep to do its job well.

Cleansing and rejuvenating your liver involve incorporating specific foods into your diet that are more gentle on the liver, such as cooked high-water vegetables (e.g., butternut squash). If you choose to eliminate meat, it is important to substitute food options that contain protein and iron so your body doesn't miss out on the benefit of these nutrients. Various herbs and spices, such as turmeric, mint, ginger, and cardamom, can also help stimulate and promote digestion. The goal is to jump-start a sluggish liver, maintain microbial diversity, and help cleanse the bowels. It may seem overwhelming at first, but it is important to balance the attention of caring for our internal support system with that of our external appearance.

DETOXIFICATION RECIPES

BASIC DETOX TEA

Ingredients:

- 1 teaspoon cumin seeds
- 1/2 teaspoon coriander seeds
- 1 cinnamon or licorice stick
- 10 fresh basil leaves
- Water, preferably filtered
- 1/2 fresh lemon

Instructions:

1. Place all ingredients (except lemon) in a medium-size sauce pan with 4 cups of filtered water.
2. Bring the water to a boil and maintain for 5 minutes.
3. Turn off heat and steep for 2–5 minutes.
4. While the tea steeps, add lemon juice by squeezing from 1/2 lemon.
5. Strain into a teapot or thermos to use throughout the day.

Makes 4 cups.

LIVER DETOX HEALTH DRINK

Ingredients:

- 1/4 tablespoon lemon juice
- 1/4 tablespoon maple syrup
- 2 liters water, preferably filtered
- 1/2 cup chopped mint
- 1/4 teaspoon cardamom powder
- 1/4 teaspoon turmeric powder

Instructions:

1. Place all ingredients (using only 1/2 liter of water) in a container and stir until well mixed.
2. Add 1/2 liter of water and steep for 10 minutes.
3. Add the remaining liter of water and mix well.
4. Drink throughout the day as needed, or per the detox instruction.

Makes 8 cups.

BUTTERNUT SQUASH APPLE SOUP

Ingredients:

- 1 teaspoon ghee
- 1 yellow onion, chopped
- 1 carrot, chopped
- 1 rib of celery, chopped
- 16 ounces butternut squash, chopped
- 3 green apples, peeled and chopped
- 1/2 teaspoon grated ginger
- 2 cups apple juice
- 1/4 teaspoon turmeric powder
- 3 cups water
- Pinches of nutmeg, cinnamon, salt, and pepper

Instructions:

1. Combine ghee, onion, carrot, and most of the celery in a saucepan. Cook over a medium heat for 5 minutes.
2. Add squash, apples, grated ginger, apple juice, turmeric, and water. Bring to a boil. Simmer for 15 minutes or until squash is soft.
3. Puree.
4. Add spices to taste.
5. Top with remaining chopped celery before serving.

Makes 4 servings.

MUNG LENTIL RICE SOUP

Ingredients:

- 3/4 cup mung dal (mung lentils), soaked in water for 1/2 hour, then drained
- 1/2 cup basmati rice, washed, soaked in water for 1/2 hour, then drained
- 1 teaspoon ginger, grated
- 1/2 teaspoon turmeric powder
- 1 tablespoon ghee
- 10 cups water
- 1 teaspoon salt
- 1 tablespoon cilantro, chopped
- lime juice

Instructions:

1. Combine the soaked and drained mung dal and rice with the ginger, turmeric, ghee, and water.
2. Boil for 45 minutes.
3. Add salt to taste if necessary.
4. Garnish with chopped cilantro and lime juice.

Makes 2 servings.

HERBAL TEA (WITH VARIATIONS)

To aid your body as you do a liver detox, drink an herbal tea at any time of the day or evening. Steep 1 teaspoon each of mint, rosemary, oregano, cilantro, sage, and basil in 4 cups of hot (175 F or preferred temperature) water. Peppermint, chamomile, and ginger tea are also good choices for a liver detox.

KHICHDI

In addition to the recipe for *khichdi* provided on page 110, there are many other ways to make this simple dish, which is recommended to prepare the body for cleansing. Let's start with the three main types of *khichdi* that ignite your digestion. The type is based on the water content, which changes the consistency from watery to broth (like soup) or thick like mashed potatoes. In Indian culture, *khichdi* is one of the first solid foods eaten by infants.

Below are the proportions of rice, split mung beans, and vegetables with the varying levels of water. Different types of rice can also be used, such as jasmine, brown, or basmati.

The split mung beans must be soaked for at least one hour before cooking.

Watery: 1 part rice, split mung beans, and vegetables
   to 8 parts water

Broth/Soup: 1 part rice, split mung beans, and vegetables
   to 6 parts water

Thick: 1 part rice, split mung beans, and vegetables
   to 4 parts water

LIVER REJUVENATION

DAY ONE

- Wake up at sunrise and find a quiet spot to ease into simple breathwork.
- Breathe through 20 cycles of inhaling and exhaling through the nose.
- Shift into 30 minutes of full-body gentle stretching.
- Notice how your body feels, both inside and out.
- Spend 15 minutes acknowledging the effort in thought or writing in a journal.
- Drink 12 ounces of lukewarm water after you finish.
- Apply warm coconut oil all over your body, letting it soak in for about 30 minutes.
- Rinse off with warm water.
- Drink a liver detox drink whenever you feel hungry or thirsty until 3:00 p.m.
- At 3:00 p.m., 5:00 p.m., and 7:00 p.m., drink a cup of hot butternut squash soup.
- Between those times, and after 7:00 p.m., drink only water and herbal teas.

DAY TWO

- Repeat the procedure above, but instead of butternut squash soup, drink the mung lentil rice soup.

DAY THREE

- Repeat the procedure on the previous page, but include soft foods after 3:00 p.m.
- Enjoy oatmeal with water, raisins, almonds, maple syrup, or honey.
- Eat fruits of different colors, like apples, pears, oranges, and berries, until 5:00 p.m.
- After 5:00 p.m. when hungry, eat the *khichdi*.
- Between the times when you eat soft foods, continue to drink the herbal tea and water.

SPIRALING

HEALING INSIDE OUTWARD

SPIRALING IS A natural form of growth. In ancient times, spirals represented ways to explore and ponder important questions; one such practice is to meditate while walking a labyrinth. I liken spiraling to the natural change that takes place in nature, such as trees expanding from the inside out. More rings equal more years of growth. Coming full circle time and time again represents a form of spiraling that is quite healing, too. I enter into new rings filled with joy leaving behind some of those "rings" that were filled with heaviness—like experiencing the unexpected death of my sister. I was spiraling, for sure, yet I had no idea about the healing that was happening as I navigated through all of it.

Spiraling is not catastrophic. In fact, while it may feel disorienting, it may just be the best thing that happens to you, even if you don't realize it in the moment. Think of the beauty of spiraling when you are experiencing a major transition or change, feel stuck in a pattern that holds you back, or feel there is more to life and something is missing in yours.

Recognizing that spiraling is a positive and natural part of growth may help you accelerate your personal growth plan. This is where it can be fun to get a little creative in our journaling or ways we solve problems. All this growth requires taking time to rejuvenate, so keep your balance, along with a sense of humor.

CLARISSA LIEBERMAN

I am an early riser and always try to wake up before my young twins in order to practice my daily rituals. If I am not running around after them, I'm working on my skin-care business, running, cycling, taking a yoga class, or cooking. I am always on the lookout for natural ways to enhance my skin-care brand. It's not just about what is applied to the skin on the outside but about loving your skin from the inside out, too. I believe in a holistic approach to glowing skin, given that balance emerges from the beautiful connection of our body, mind, and soul. My discipline of a daily routine brings significant balance to my life. I go to bed at 10:00 p.m. and get up at 6:00 a.m. *Nidra*, which is the physiological state of rest, meaning sleep, is a priority, as I know that eight hours of sleep helps my skin look its best. It enhances *ojas*, the connector of mind, body, and soul, bringing balance in its purest form.

Getting up earlier than my twins is definitely a test of my dedication. I find myself creeping into the bathroom before they are awake. I drink a lot of water every day, which helps me maintain clear skin, but I recently switched to warm water between meals, as drinking with food can interrupt the digestive fire, compromising optimal digestion. My *Pitta* digestion (*Pitta* is a dosha type that is often fiery) can become very acidic when I'm out of balance, leading to inflammation that shows up on my skin. My skin rituals have always been important, some-

thing I learned by observing my mother, but what became really important is using toxin-free, plant-derived
skin-care regimens.

Abhyanga facial massage is one of the most important rituals for me, given the dry condition of my skin,
but also to help eliminate toxins, naturally firm and lift
the skin, and stimulate the blood flow to the skin surface. I practice the ritual at least twice a week (see Glowing Skin pg 162). All of this knowledge encourages me to
show up every day, no matter what is happening in my
life. Taking care of my body is how I can best show up as
my best self for my family. Learning to be in a relation-
ship with Ayurveda [can become] a love affair—a relation-
ship that changes over time as you grow and learn more
about yourself and what balances your mind, body, and
soul every day.

GLOWING SKIN

THOUGHT BUBBLE:

"I need balance in my life for myself and for my family."

SIMPLE ANCIENT RITUAL:

- Mix 1/4 teaspoon tumeric powder with 1 tablespoon of chickpea flour.
- Make a paste by adding almond oil, water, or milk, depending on your skin type:
- If your skin is dry, add 1 teaspoon of almond oil, followed by a little water until the consistency desired is achieved.
- If your skin is sensitive, add only milk.
- If your skin is oily, add only water.
- Apply the paste onto individual body parts or all over your body.
- Relax for 15–20 minutes until the paste fully dries.

MASTERY QUOTE:

"What I dream of is an art of balance."
—*Henri Matisse*

MODERN TAKE:

Herbal cleansing prepares the skin for self-massage by opening up the pores. The herbal paste can be used in place of soap for your regular routine as it removes both bacteria and the by-products of perspiration. It stimulates the skin tissue for a healthier, more glowing complexion. Another way to utilize cleansing is for a seasonal detox, a staple for holistic health. When the seasons are in transition, try a one- to two-day cleanse of herbal teas, fruit juices, cleansing herbs, and warming soups to cleanse the body. The cleanse removes any buildup of toxins that have accumulated due to weak or compromised digestion and poor diet. It is like a reset at the beginning of the season to allow the body to perform at its best. Ayurveda teaches self-love, self-realization, acceptance, and understanding. Listen to your body, and give it what it needs every day.

DISCOVER MORE:

skin toning; *platza*; icthyotherapy; *hamman*; *suna-mushi*

REJUVENATING BATH

THOUGHT BUBBLE:

"My muscles ache. I need to soak in the tub."

SIMPLE ANCIENT RITUAL:

- Use the body paste (see Glowing Skin, page 162), then gently brush it off with a towel.
- Massage the body with warmed sesame oil mixed with 1 teaspoon of tumeric powder.
- Take a warm bath for 15-20 minutes.
- Before getting into the tub, add the following, depending on your skin type:
    - For dry skin, add a tablespoon of honey and 10 drops of rosewater.
    - For oily skin, add 10 drops of lavender or lemon oil.
    - For sensitive skin, add 1/2 cup of dry milk powder.

MASTERY QUOTE:

"We must always change, renew, rejuvenate ourselves; otherwise, we harden."
—Johann Wolfgang von Goethe

MODERN TAKE:

Taking a nice, long bath with candles and salts allows me to bring some welcomed comfort to my body. There is nothing like that wonderful feeling of dipping into warm water and allowing my body and mind to relax; adding Epsom salts to the bath is also great for sore muscles after a full day laboring over the computer and running errands. Bathing in water has long been a ritual for care and relaxation. The Greeks and Romans even built elaborate bathhouses that could accommodate thousands of people at any one time. Times have changed, of course, given the evolution of religion, privacy, and modern plumbing. However, spas, saunas, birthing pools, hot springs, and mineral baths all still have their place in practicing good health and seeking out ways to decompress and lower stress.

DISCOVER MORE:

skin toning; *platza*; icthyotherapy; *hamman*; *suna-mushi*

HAIKU POEM

THOUGHT BUBBLE:

"I want my journaling time to be more creative and fun."

SIMPLE ANCIENT RITUAL:
- Write 3-5 sentences describing one of your wishes (e.g., a dream vacation).
- Use words related to the senses—sight, hearing, touch, smell, and taste (e.g., "juicy").
- Write one or two more sentences that are unrelated to your wish but that describe something you enjoy.
- Now pick out the pithy phrases from all of your writing that grab your attention.
- Count the number of syllables within each phrase.
- Modify the phrases so that they contain either five or seven syllables—and don't overthink this step.
- Begin structuring the poem as follows: Three lines, with five syllables in the first line, seven syllables in the second line, and five syllables in the third line.
- Think about the combination of these phrases, and see what new ideas emerge.
- Rewrite the poem using the stand-alone 5-7-5 haiku format and smile.

"The wheel is come full circle."
—William Shakespeare

MODERN TAKE:

Haiku is a form of Japanese poetry that uses seventeen syllables to capture a moment and create an image in the reader's mind. Think of it as a small opening that leads you into a magical dream world. A typical haiku focuses on a season (like springtime) and chooses words that suggest that time of year (such as *tulips*). A division in the poem can create surprising relationships, and emotions can come through the sensorial description of the scene you depict. Ultimately, crafting a haiku like this can spark new ideas and even become an inspiration for achieving personal goals. Here's an example of one I wrote:

I am a tall tree
now spiraling to new heights
rooted in the now

my limbs signal growth
each spiral is different
until finally

living full circle
rainbows igniting dancing
I recognize me

DISCOVER MORE:

haiku; creative writing; journaling; poetry slams; Matsuo Basho

LIVING FULL CIRCLE

I am truly living full circle—both professionally and personally. What I mean by *professionally* is that I am reframing and expanding upon the foundational education that underpinned my graduate degrees in both food science and nutrition. My intent is to advance the thinking behind product development in order to integrate what we now know about the holistic needs of an individual—because solely focusing on the functional benefits of products has done us a disservice.

Lifestyle medicine experts generally focus on six evidenced-based approaches, including whole foods, plant-based diets, regular physical activity, adequate sleep, stress management, and avoidance of risky substances—all to reverse, prevent, and treat chronic disease. But while calling out stress management as a specific area of focus is important, we do not focus enough on the "hidden stress" and all the challenges that accompany the environments we inhabit.

What I mean by *personally* is that I am reexamining how I spend my time and where I place my attention. I will not perpetuate the accumulation of stress, which acts to repress my basic needs of being human. Borrowing from the construct of the rituals

I have shared in this field guide, here are a few questions to help you explore and expunge hidden stress:

- What is grounded? Do I know and recognize what that feels like?
- Am I mobilizing or stalling growth?
- What are my blind spots? Can I accept the cranky wheels?
- Am I signaling positive change with my actions?
- Am I sensing where I am stuck?
- Am I holding on to the past?
- Am I uncovering hidden barriers in order to move forward?
- Am I designing my day so that I can flow and easily shift where needed?
- Am I taking care to zone my energetic spaces and place boundaries when needed?
- Am I transitioning and welcoming more hopeful serendipity?
- Am I practicing the values that I want to embody?
- Am I owning the energy I put out into the world?
- Am I noticing the change around me and observing the ripple effect?
- Am I spiraling up and acknowledging the healing that is happening?
- Am I accepting who I am? Am I accepting others?
- Am I accepting what others can and cannot see?
- Am I feeling better?

These are just a few questions to probe as you practice and reflect on the rituals. I hope you use the journal pages in the back of this book to explore these ideas further and jot down additional questions that surface—all to enhance your commitment to remove stress and feel better, too. While a healthy lifestyle can certainly improve our overall health, the word *lifestyle* does not offer specific direction that can be personalized. Taking the time to ask and answer these kinds of questions in a journal that you can pick up and reread anytime can bring forward fresh insight for how best to take care of both your body and your mind.

There can be a disconnect between what we think we know and how we apply that to our everyday lives. Think about the major changes you have made in your lifestyle with food and exercise and how that may not holistically support the flow of your energetic zones. As an extreme example, the energetic nature of everything we touch sometimes gets overlooked when we select the food we eat, or when and even where we eat it—at a table with friends or in a car on the way to a meeting. Biting into a crisp apple just picked off the tree is energetically different than eating those apples hidden in the cobbler on the TV tray dinner in two gulps. All of this is to say that we can overlook the more basic aspects of our lifestyle that can undermine our goals for better health and less stress.

The focus of this guide is on small things that you can do every day to positively impact your well-being. Think about your body as a container that works hard every day in order for you to enjoy the things you need and want to do. What you put in your body matters, including texture that is accessible for digestion, composition that supports your need for nutrients, and energetic value. If you are experiencing some kind of major transition or a lot of change that increases stress, that also affects how well your body can function. If you feel stuck in a pattern that holds you back, then explore ways to unblock those energy zones. Certain life circumstances, like the loss of a loved one, will create unclear or confusing experiences that require you to take more time for yourself to work through the loss and grief. In addition, if you are accelerating your own personal growth path, you may be shifting into areas that make you feel uncomfortable, including managing relationships that are no longer healthy. In any case, let breathwork ground and reground you until it becomes a natural reaction to any stress you may encounter.

I have learned what I need to do in order to shift to and sustain feeling good. It is not always the easiest choice. Wellness may be a commodity in our society, but not at the expense of my own personal well-being. I listen to the whispers and quiet nudges of sages who say all the answers are within me. Yes, there will always be an endless sea of stuff to buy and try, but rip all the fluff away and identify what you truly need and want. Unplug and take a walk. Eat root vegetables and mushy foods to reset your digestion. Drink warm water to help your energy flow. Make room for just one small change, and observe if it helps you feel better.

I have spent decades exploring the keys to wellness and found my answers by looking to the past. I know now that I have come full circle in believing it is up to me to bring forward better ideas—starting with the art of stress-free living. Putting together a 1,000-piece jigsaw puzzles on cardboard panels has become a modern form of my occasional evening meditation. Find your own version for getting clear so serendipity can arrive with new adventures and surprising invitations. Maybe start by creating a simple haiku and see where the fun leads.

Come back to you—that's all that matters.

ACKNOWLEDGMENTS

My heartfelt gratitude goes out to the many who have showered me with love and encouragement while translating and honoring the rituals expressed in this book. The entire process was its own gift—hundreds of creative experiences that unfolded in order to unleash the wisdom of the past through the hearts of old souls who remain hopeful about tomorrow.

Thank you, Dr. Naina Marballi and your staff, for your dedication to Ayurveda World and for keeping alive the mastery of ancient wisdom while bringing practical healing into the world. Thank you to the entire holistic healing certification class of 2018–2019 for being willing to get "on the mat" and start fresh time and time again. I am grateful for the bonds that we formed as we circled up to soak in the lessons, ask endless questions, and keep our sense of humor while we witnessed such personal transformations. I am grateful for Daria, Jessica, Nikki, Lina, Jayne, Clarissa, Julia, and Maryanne for their courageous stands and for agreeing to share in this book a snapshot of their personal story, given the ways that ancient wisdom has changed their lives. They give new meaning to what it means to "walk the talk."

Thank you, Brianna, for helping me keep it real; your incredible story of love and loss is inspirational to me and your knowing of what truly helps make health and wellness advise feel less like judgment has given me invaluable insight.

This book would not have been possible without the bold vision and wisdom of Theresa DiMasi and her talented crew at Tiller—Sam, Kate, Anja, Matt, Lauren, and others—who are all focused on giving a louder voice to culturally relevant stories in a more timely and comprehensive way. Thank you, Lauren, for making the role of editor look easy while enabling these rituals to sing and dance into the world.

Thank you to my entire family for their support, encouragement, and confidence in me in light of all that we have experienced and endured. I am especially grateful for my mom and dad, my prayer warriors, who are constantly in tune to my weather vane.

Mostly, I am grateful for my soulful children, Madi and Keaton, and hope the insight in this book keeps alive my wish for them to experience a life of feeling good while surrounded by love and laughter as they forge the path that is uniquely theirs.

Love, peace, and patience to all—remember patience takes care of your body and mind.

Namaste.

THOUGHT BUBBLE AND MASTERY QUOTE REFERENCE GUIDE

Below is a reference guide to the "thought bubbles" and "mastery quotes" I've included throughout the pages of this field guide. Think of them as prompts for choosing an ancient ritual. This list can offer quick access to match what you need with practices that support it. The thought bubbles alongside the mastery quotes may also spark ideas for you to write about on your journal pages or stimulate you to search out ways to extend and personalize your path toward reducing stress and feeling better.

GROUNDING

Breath IQ

THOUGHT BUBBLE:

"There are so many distractions, I cannot focus!"

MASTERY QUOTE:

"When the breath is still, so is the mind." —The Hatha Yoga Pradīpikā

Breath Scan

THOUGHT BUBBLE:

"What is the correct way to breathe— through my nose or my mouth?"

MASTERY QUOTE:

"Great things are done by a series of small things brought together." —*Vincent van Gogh*

Alternate Nostril Breathing (ANB)

THOUGHT BUBBLE:

"I can hardly breathe. I feel panicky."

MASTERY QUOTE:

"If we take care of the minutes, the years will take care of themselves."
—Benjamin Franklin

Clean Slate

THOUGHT BUBBLE:

"I have too much on my plate, and the day hasn't even started!"

MASTERY QUOTE:

"Poetry is breathing words that give a reader pause."
—Ankita Singhal

Daybreak

THOUGHT BUBBLE:

"I need some peace and quiet in my life."

MASTERY QUOTE:

"It is well to be up before daybreak, for such habits contribute to health, wealth, and wisdom."
—Aristotle

MOBILIZING

Joint Scan

THOUGHT BUBBLE:

"My stiff fingers and knees keep me from doing things I enjoy."

MASTERY QUOTE:

"Little by little, one travels far."
—Spanish proverb

Speaking Up

THOUGHT BUBBLE:

"Why don't I just say something?"

MASTERY QUOTE:

"There is no greater agony than bearing an untold story inside you."
—Maya Angelou

Belly Jump-Start

THOUGHT BUBBLE:

"I sit most of the day and cannot stay regular!"

MASTERY QUOTE:

"I've had it with you and your emotional constipation."
—Washington Irving

Mobilizing Resilience

THOUGHT BUBBLE:

"My feet are tired and hurt after a long day."

MASTERY QUOTE:

"At the end of the day, let there be no excuses, no explanations, no regrets."

—Steve Maraboli

SIGNALING

Self-Assurance Hand Gesture

THOUGHT BUBBLE:

"Why do I keep second-guessing myself? I know I can do it."

MASTERY QUOTE:

"They are not exercises, but techniques which place the physical body in positions that cultivate awareness, relaxation, concentration, and meditation."

—Swami Satyananda Saraswati

Acceptance Hand Gesture

THOUGHT BUBBLE:

"I feel really sad and cannot seem to shake it."

MASTERY QUOTE:

"Acceptance doesn't mean resignation; it means understanding that something is what it is and that there's got to be a way through it."

—Michael J. Fox

Self-Confidence Hand Gesture

THOUGHT BUBBLE:

"I am tired of holding back and not speaking up."

MASTERY QUOTE:

"A man cannot be comfortable without his own approval."

—Mark Twain

Grounding Hand Gesture

THOUGHT BUBBLE:

"I feel so frenzied and just need to get a grip."

MASTERY QUOTE:

"All the art of living lies in a fine mingling of letting go and holding on."

—Henry Havelock Ellis

Patience Hand Gesture

THOUGHT BUBBLE:

"I am so sleep deprived, I am easily triggered and upset."

MASTERY QUOTE:

"Patience is a virtue."

—Proverb

SENSING

Tongue IQ

THOUGHT BUBBLE:

"My tongue feels thick. Yuck!"

MASTERY QUOTE:

"The body never lies."

—Mae West

Palms Up

THOUGHT BUBBLE:

"Another deep breath? I think I am going to lose it!"

MASTERY QUOTE:

"When anger arises, think of the consequences."

—Confucius

Finger Tapping

THOUGHT BUBBLE:

"The pain is so bad; I am desperate for relief."

MASTERY QUOTE:

"The latest research has shown when we tap on the endpoints of meridians in the body, we send a calming signal to the amygdala (the fight-or-flight center) in the brain."

—Nick Ortner, from an interview with The Connecticut Post *(May 25, 2013)*

Self-Massage

THOUGHT BUBBLE:

"My neck is stiff, and my jaw feels tight."

MASTERY QUOTE:

"A gentle touch is all it takes to tame the wildest of men."

—Anthony T. Hincks

Warming Up

THOUGHT BUBBLE:

"I feel so cold; I can't warm up."

MASTERY QUOTE:

"There is no illusion greater than fear."

—Lao Tzu, Tao Te Ching

Tranquil Shower

THOUGHT BUBBLE:

"As a new mom, I want to keep life in balance without disregarding my own needs."

MASTERY QUOTE:

"Youth fades; love droops; the leaves of friendship fall; a mother's secret hope outlives them all."
—Oliver Wendell Holmes

ZONING

Red or R-Zone

THOUGHT BUBBLE:

"I am so upset. I cannot believe this is happening."

MASTERY QUOTE:

"Everything we experience— no matter how unpleasant—comes into our lives to teach us something."
—Iyanla Vanzant

Orange or O-Zone

THOUGHT BUBBLE:

"I am so uninspired . . . listless, whatever."

MASTERY QUOTE:

"The person who sends out positive thoughts activates the world around him positively and draws back to himself positive results."
—Norman Vincent Peale

Yellow or Y-Zone

THOUGHT BUBBLE:

"I do not like who I am right now."

MASTERY QUOTE:

"I must be willing to give up what I am in order to become what I will be."
—Albert Einstein

Green or G-Zone

THOUGHT BUBBLE:

"I want to be more optimistic about the future."

MASTERY QUOTE:

"The future belongs to those who believe in the beauty of their dreams."
—Eleanor Roosevelt

Blue or B-Zone

THOUGHT BUBBLE:

"I am constantly apologizing! But for what?"

MASTERY QUOTE:

"It took me quite a long time to develop a voice, and now that I have it, I am not going to be silent."
—Madeleine K. Albright

Indigo or I-Zone

THOUGHT BUBBLE:

"I just need to trust my gut and make a decision."

MASTERY QUOTE:

"There is deep wisdom within our very flesh, if we can only come to our senses and feel it."
—Elizabeth A. Behnke

Violet or V-Zone

THOUGHT BUBBLE:

"I feel disconnected from everything happening in my life."

MASTERY QUOTE:

"The best thing you could do is master the chaos in you. You are not thrown into the fire; you are the fire."
—Mama Indigo

Quiet Zone

THOUGHT BUBBLE:

"I feel frazzled and need time to think."

MASTERY QUOTE:

"Be silent. That heart speaks without tongue or lips."
—Rumi

Good Vibe Poem

THOUGHT BUBBLE:

"I need to shake myself out of this rut!"

MASTERY QUOTE:

"You are precisely as big as what you love and precisely as small as what you allow to annoy you."
—Robert Anton Wilson

Re-Zone

THOUGHT BUBBLE:

"There is so much clutter, it is weighing me down."

MASTERY QUOTE:

"Clutter is not just physical stuff; it's old ideas, toxic relationships, and bad habits."
—Eleanor Brown

Judge-Free Zone

THOUGHT BUBBLE:

"I am responsible for the energy I put out in the world and for the energy I choose to take in."

MASTERY QUOTE:

"Every time you smile at someone, it is an action of love, a gift to that person, a beautiful thing."
—Mother Teresa

SHIFTING

A.M. Wake-Up Call

THOUGHT BUBBLE:

"I feel so rushed in the morning."

MASTERY QUOTE:

"Early to bed and early to rise makes a man healthy, wealthy, and wise."
—Proverb

Tongue Scraping

THOUGHT BUBBLE:

"My breath smells disgusting in the morning."

MASTERY QUOTE:

"A man too busy to take care of his health is like a mechanic too busy to take care of his tools."
—Spanish proverb

Oil Pulling

THOUGHT BUBBLE:

"I've brushed my teeth, but is the inside of my mouth really clean?"

MASTERY QUOTE: *"*

They sure are handy when you smile, so keep your teeth around a while."
    —Dr. Seuss

TRANSITIONING

Break I Fast

THOUGHT BUBBLE:

"I want to wake up and feel energized for the day."

MASTERY QUOTE:

"Often when you think you're at the end of something, you're at the beginning of something else."
—Fred Rogers

Preparing a Pot of *Khichdi*

THOUGHT BUBBLE:

"I don't have time to prepare wholesome meals every day."

MASTERY QUOTE:

"One cannot think well, love well, sleep well, if one has not dined well."
—Virginia Woolf

Warm Golden Milk

THOUGHT BUBBLE:

"I love a nightly ritual, but I don't want to drink alcohol."

MASTERY QUOTE:

"The way you prepare the bed, so shall you sleep."
 —Yiddish proverb

Cumin Coriander Fennel (CCF) Tea Break

THOUGHT BUBBLE:

"I feel so heavy and bloated."

MASTERY QUOTE:

"Drinking a daily cup of tea will surely starve the apothecary."
—Ancient Chinese proverb

Silence Is Golden

THOUGHT BUBBLE:

"I can barely function, and I just want to crawl into bed."

MASTERY QUOTE:

"The only person you are destined to become is the person you decide to be."
—Ralph Waldo Emerson

PRACTICING

Caterpillar

THOUGHT BUBBLE:

"I need to do something physical to help me wind down at night."

MASTERY QUOTE:

"The body benefits from movement, and the mind benefits from stillness."
—Sakyong Mipham

Gratitude Journal

THOUGHT BUBBLE:

"Nothing went my way today!"

MASTERY QUOTE:

"Gratitude is a powerful catalyst for happiness. It's the spark that lights a fire of joy in your soul."
—Amy Collette

Prayer Chain

THOUGHT BUBBLE:

"My friend is in serious trouble and needs support."

MASTERY QUOTE:

"Heaven is full of answers to prayer for which no one ever bothered to ask."
—Billy Graham

Private Dance Party

THOUGHT BUBBLE:

"My body wants to dance, but I don't feel like getting dressed and going out with friends."

MASTERY QUOTE:

"Dance is the hidden language of the soul."
—Martha Graham

Nature Walk

THOUGHT BUBBLE:

"I rarely get to play on the grass or take a walk in the woods."

MASTERY QUOTE:

"The clearest way into the Universe is through a forest wilderness."
—John Muir

OWNING

EMF Detox

THOUGHT BUBBLE:

"I can't fall asleep. Then when I do, I wake up throughout the night."

MASTERY QUOTE:

"Rest and be thankful."
—William Wadsworth

Sunset Fast

THOUGHT BUBBLE:

"I think it is time to rethink my daily routine."

MASTERY QUOTE:

"Whenever you find yourself on the side of the majority, it's time to pause and reflect."
—Mark Twain

Quick Fast

THOUGHT BUBBLE:

"I have not been taking the time to eat as well as I normally do."

MASTERY QUOTE:

"When you change the way you look at things, the things you look at change."
—Max Planck

One-Day Fast

THOUGHT BUBBLE:

"I need to give my body a break."

MASTERY QUOTE:

"Take care of your body. It's the only place you have to live."
—Jim Rohn

Haiku Poem

THOUGHT BUBBLE:

"I want my journaling time to be more creative and fun."

MASTERY QUOTE:

"The wheel is come full circle."
—William Shakespeare

SPIRALING

Glowing Skin

THOUGHT BUBBLE:

"I need balance in my life for myself and for my family."

MASTERY QUOTE:

"What I dream of is an art of balance."
—Henri Matisse

Rejuvenating Bath

THOUGHT BUBBLE:

"My muscles ache. I need to soak in the tub."

MASTERY QUOTE:

"We must always change, renew, rejuvenate ourselves; otherwise, we harden."
—Johann Wolfgang von Goethe

INDEX

A

abdomen, 4, 6, 45, 58, 96
  belly jump-start and,
    24-25
acceptance, xix, xxv, 37, 50,
    88, 98, 163, 170
  acceptance hand
    gestures, 34-35
Albright, Madeleine K., 75
ancient rituals:
  format of, xxvii-xxix
  themes of, xxxi-xxxii
  what you need for, xxx
Angelou, Maya, 22
apples, 114, 155, 171
  butternut squash apple
    soup, 151
Aristotle, 14
aromas, xviii-xix, 7, 100, 114,
    135, 166
  sensing and, 44,
    53-57, 59
  zoning and, 67, 69, 71, 73,
    75, 77, 79
Ayurveda, xix, xxiv, 13, 28,
    39, 140
  sensing and, 46-47, 49,
    53, 57, 59
  shifting and, 93, 95-96,
    99, 101
  spiraling and, 161, 163

B

Babine, Jayne, 57
balance, xiii-xiv, xix,
    xxiii-xxiv, xxxii, 64, 83,
    121, 149
  grounding and, 2, 5, 9, 11,
    39, 42
  noticing flows and, 135, 145
  sensing and, 44, 46-47,
    53, 57-58

shifting and, 93, 95-96
  spiraling and, 159-62
bathing, 55, 87, 121, 131, 160
  rejuvenating bath, 164-65
Behnke, Elizabeth A., 77
body, 31, 33, 106, 171
  grounding and, 9, 11, 14-15,
    39, 122
  liver rejuvenation and, 149,
    153-54
  mobilizing and, 19, 27-28
  noticing flows and, 134-36,
    138, 141-42, 144
  routines and, 121-22, 128
  sensing and, 45-47, 49-51,
    58-59
  shifting and, 93-96
  spiraling and, 163-65
  zoning and, 64-65, 67, 87
  see also mind-body
    connection
brain, 95, 98, 122, 165, 171
  grounding and, 2, 10-11
  noticing flows and, 135-36, 144
  sensing and, 45, 51, 54
  transitioning and, 106, 115
  zoning and, 65-66, 68, 70-72,
    74, 76-78
  see also mind-body
    connection
breakfasts, 13-14, 96-97, 106-9
  break | fast, 108-9
breath, breathwork, xviii-xix,
    xxiv, xxix, 19, 41, 47,
    130, 144
  alternate nostril breathing
    (ANB), 3, 8-9
  breath IQ, 4-5, 7
  breath scan, 6-7
  clean slate and, 10-11
  daybreak and, 14-15
  grounding and, 2-15, 95, 122,
    172
  liver rejuvenation and, 149,
    154

shifting and, 95, 100-101
  zoning and, 66, 68, 70, 72, 74,
    76, 78, 80-81
Brown, Eleanor, 84
butternut squash, 149
  butternut squash apple
    soup, 151
  butternut squash soup, 154

C

Calonge, Nikki, 28
coconut oil, xxx, 20, 26, 154
  sensing and, 52, 54, 58
  shifting and, 94-96, 102-3
  transitioning and, 110-13
Collette, Amy, 124
commitment, xiv, xix-xx, xxx,
    87, 135, 170
confidence, 23, 32-33, 106
  self-confidence hand
    gesture, 36-37
  zoning and, 67, 71, 75
Confucius, 49
constipation, 19, 24-25, 39
coriander, 110-11, 150
  cumin coriander fennel
    (CCF) tea break, 114-15
cumin, 110, 113-15, 150
  cumin coriander fennel
    (CCF) tea break, 114-15
Cygan, Jessica, 13

D

dance, dancing, xiii, 28, 87, 121,
    167
  private dance party, 128-29
detoxification, 93, 97, 111, 123, 163
  basic detox tea, 150
  detoxification recipes, xxx,
    150-53
  EMF detox, 138-39
  liver detox health drink,
    150-51
  noticing flows and, 136-39,
    145

digestion, 39, 58, 95, 171–72
liver rejuvenation and, 149, 153
mobilizing and, 19, 24–25
noticing flows and, 134–35,
143
sensing and, 45–47
spiraling and, 160, 163
transitioning and, 111, 114–15
discovering more, xxvii, xxix
grounding and, 5, 7, 9, 11, 15
hand gestures and, 33, 35,
37, 39, 41
mobilizing and, 21, 23, 25, 27
noticing flows and, 139, 141,
143, 145
routines and, 123, 125, 127, 129
sensing and, 47, 49, 51, 53,
55, 59
shifting and, 99, 101, 103
spiraling and, 163, 165, 167
transitioning and, 109, 111, 113,
115, 117
zoning and, 67, 69, 71, 73, 75,
77, 79, 81, 83, 85, 89

E

Einstein, Albert, 71
electromagnetic fields (EMFs),
135–39
EMF detox, 138–39
Ellis, Henry Havelock, 39
Emerson, Ralph Waldo, 116
emotions, xv, xx–xxi, xxiii, 2–3,
24, 94, 109, 129, 167
hand gestures and, 31, 34–35,
37
noticing flows and, 134–35
sensing and, 50–51
zoning and, 63, 66, 68–70, 72,
74, 76–78, 80, 84, 87
energy, energy management,
xviii, xxiii–xxv, xxviii–xxx, 9,
109, 170–72
hand gestures and, 31, 33,
39, 42

mobilizing and, 19, 26–27
noticing flows and, 134–37
routines and, 121, 127, 129
sensing and, 45, 49, 51, 53,
57, 59
shifting and, 96–97
zoning and, xxx, 63–79, 83–89,
170
eyes, 50, 52
zoning and, 64, 66, 68, 70, 72,
74, 76, 78, 80

F

fasts, fasting:
break | fast, 108–9
intermittent fasting (IF), 117,
141–43, 145
noticing flows and, 134–35,
138, 140–44
one-day fast, 144–45
quick fast, 142–43
sunset fast, 140–41
feng shui, 84–85
fennel, 102
cumin coriander fennel
(CCF) tea break, 114–15
fingers, 20–21, 125
finger tapping, 50–51
hand gestures and, 31–32, 34,
36, 38, 40
sensing and, 48–52
Fox, Michael J., 35
Franklin, Benjamin, 8
fruits, 47, 75, 77, 114, 151, 155, 163

G

ghee, xxx, 97, 151–52
ginger, 121
liver rejuvenation and, 149,
151–52
transitioning and, 108, 110–12
Goethe, Johann Wolfgang
von, 164
golden milk, 112–13, 121
Graham, Billy, 126

Graham, Martha, 128
gratitude, xxxi, 121, 130, 138
gratitude journal, 124–25
shifting and, 96–97
grounding, 2–15, 42, 170
alternate nostril breathing
(ANB) and, 3, 8–9
ancient rituals and,
xxxi–xxxii, 3–4, 6, 8,
10–11, 14, 95
breathing and, 2–15, 95, 122,
172
breath IQ and, 4–5, 7
breath scan and, 6–7
clean slate and, 10–11
daybreak and, 14–15
grounding hand gesture,
38–39

H

hands, hand gestures, xxv, 28,
31–42
acceptance hand gestures,
34–35
ancient rituals and, xxxii,
31–32, 34, 36, 38, 40
grounding hand gesture,
38–39
palms up and, 48–49
patience hand gesture,
40–41
self-assurance hand gesture,
32–33
self-confidence hand
gesture, 36–37
sensing and, 44–49, 54
stress and, 2, 170
Hatha Yoga Pradīpikā, the, 4
heart, xvi, xxiv, 2, 72–73, 80,
149
herbs, 140, 145, 163
liver rejuvenation and, 149,
152, 154–55
shifting and, 93, 96–97
transitioning and, 108, 113, 115

Hincks, Anthony T., 52
holistic health, xiii, xv–xvi,
    xix–xxi, xxv, xxxi, 28,
    42, 129, 144, 169, 171
  sensing and, 44, 53
  shifting and, 93–94
  spiraling and, 160, 163
  transitioning and, 106–7, 113
Holmes, Oliver Wendell, 58

I

Irving, Washington, 24

J

joints, xxiii, 31, 49, 58, 113
  joint scan, 20–21
  mobilizing and, 19–21, 27
journaling, xxx, 154, 170–71
  gratitude journal, 124–25
  noticing flows and, 144–45
  spiraling and, 159, 166–67

K

Kalinina, Daria, 93–97, 121
khichdi, 96–97
  liver rejuvenation and, 153,
    155
  recipes for, 110–11, 153

L

Lad, Vasant, 95
Lao Tzu, 54
Lieberman, Clarissa, 160–61
liver, 25, 44–45, 143, 145
  liver detox health drink,
    150–51
  rejuvenation of, xxiii, xxx,
    135, 149–55
  transitioning and, 116–17

M

Mama Indigo, 79
Maraboli, Steve, 26
Matisse, Henri, 162
meditation, xxiv, 28, 117, 159, 172

grounding and, 5, 7, 10–13
hand gestures and, 33, 35, 37,
    39, 41–42
routines and, 122, 131
shifting and, 95–96
So-Hum meditation, 10, 96
zoning and, 69, 81, 83, 87
mind–body connection, xv–xvi,
    xix–xx, xxiv–xxv, 2, 5, 13,
    160–61
Mipham, Sakyong, 122
mobilizing, 19–28, 170
  ancient rituals and, xxxii,
    19–20, 22, 24, 26
  belly jump-start and, 24–25
  joint scan and, 20–21
  mobilizing resilience, 26–27
  speaking up and, 22–23
modern takes, xxvii, xxix
  grounding and, 4–5, 7, 9–11,
    14–15
  hand gestures and, 33, 35,
    37, 39, 41
  mobilizing and, 21–27
  noticing flows and, 139–45
  routines and, 122–31
  sensing and, 46–47, 49, 51,
    53–55, 59
  shifting and, 99, 101–3
  spiraling and, 163, 165, 167
  transitioning and, 109, 111,
    113–17
  zoning and, 67, 69, 71, 73, 75,
    77, 79, 81, 83–85, 89
moods, 31, 35, 64
  sensing and, 44, 54–55
  shifting and, 93, 96–97
mornings, 28, 35, 47, 121,
    140–41
  A.M. wake-up call and,
    98–99
  break | fast and, 108–9
  grounding and, 10, 13, 15
  shifting and, 95, 97–101
  transitioning and, 108–9, 116

Mother Teresa, 88
movement, xviii, xxiv, 28, 31, 45,
    122, 128–29
  mobilizing and, 19–21
Muir, John, 130
mung lentils, mung beans,
    152–54
  mung lentil rice soup, 152,
    154
  transitioning and, 110–11, 114

N

noticing flows, 134–45, 170
  ancient rituals and, xxxii,
    136–38, 140, 142, 144
  EMF detox and, 138–39
  one-day fast and, 144–45
  quick fast and, 142–43
  sunset fast and, 140–41
nutrition, xiv–xvi, xxiii–xxv, 14,
    19, 25, 125, 169, 171–72
  liver rejuvenation and,
    149–55
  noticing flows and, 134–35,
    137, 139–43
  sensing and, 45, 47, 54–55
  shifting and, 94, 96–97
  spiraling and, 160, 163
  transitioning and, 106–16
  see also recipes

O

O'Brien, Maryanne, 137
oils, xviii, xxx, 89, 96, 121, 164
  mobilizing and, 20–21, 26
  oil pulling, 102–3
  sensing and, 44, 53–57, 59
  see also coconut oil
Ortner, Nick, 51

P

pain, xvii, 49–50, 93, 113
patience, xiii, xxix, xxxii
  patience hand gesture, 40–41
Peale, Norman Vincent, 69

personal spotlights, xxxi, 13, 28, 42, 57, 87, 121, 137
 shifting and, 93–97
 spiraling and, 160–61
Planck, Max, 142
poems, poetry, 10
 "Good Vibe Poem," 82–83
 haiku poem, 166–67, 172
prayers, praying, 13, 81, 121
 prayer chain, 126–27

R

recipes, xviii, 93, 110–14
 detoxification recipes, xxx, 150–53
 for *khichdi*, 110–11, 153
 for warm golden milk, 112–13
rejuvenation, xix–xx, 44–45, 159
 of liver, xxiii, xxx, 135, 149–55
 noticing flows and, 134–35, 145
 rejuvenating bath, 164–65
resilience, xiii, 3, 26–28
 mobilizing resilience, 26–27
rice, xxx, 152–54
 mung lentil rice soup, 152, 154
 transitioning and, 110–11
Rogers, Fred, 108
Rohn, Jim, 144
Roosevelt, Eleanor, 73
routines, xv, 35, 57, 121–31, 163, 170
 ancient rituals and, xx–xxi, xxiii, xxix, xxxi–xxxii, 122, 124, 126, 128, 130
 caterpillar and, 122–23
 gratitude journal and, 124–25
 grounding and, 14–15
 mobilizing and, 19, 21, 25
 nature walk and, 130–31
 noticing flows and, 140–41, 145
 prayer chain and, 126–27
 private dance party and, 128–29
 shifting and, 94, 97
 transitioning and, 106, 109, 113
Rumi, 80

S

Saraswati, Swami Satyananda, 33
seasons, xxx, 64, 99, 135, 163, 167
self-massage, xxx, 96
 mobilizing and, 20–21, 24–28
 sensing and, 44, 49, 52–54, 57–59
 spiraling and, 161–64
senses, sensing, xix, xxiii, 5, 7, 28, 44–59, 64, 77, 166–67, 170
 ancient rituals and, xxxii, 44, 46, 48–50, 52, 54, 58
 finger tapping and, 50–51
 palms up and, 48–49
 self-massage and, 44, 49, 52–54, 57–59
 tongue IQ and, 46–47
 tranquil shower and, 58–59
 warming up and, 54–55
Seuss, Dr., 102
Shakespeare, William, 167
shifting, xx, xxiv, xxix, 28, 31, 44, 79, 93–103, 134, 145
 A.M. wake-up call and, 98–99
 ancient rituals and, xxxii, 97–100, 102
 oil pulling and, 102–3
 stress and, 95, 98, 170, 172
 tongue scraping and, 94, 100–101
showers, showering, 83, 96, 121, 125
 sensing and, 44, 57–59
 tranquil shower, 58–59
silence, 134, 144
 shifting and, 95–96
 silence is golden, 116–17
 zoning and, 75, 79–81
Singhal, Ankita, 10
skin, 26, 34, 96
 glowing skin, 162–63

sensing and, 44, 51, 54, 58
 spiraling and, 160–65
sleep, xviii, xxiv–xxv, 21, 149, 160, 169
 grounding and, 14–15
 hand gestures and, 39–41
 noticing flows and, 136, 138–41, 145
 routines and, 121, 124
 sensing and, 44–45
 shifting and, 93–94, 98–99
 transitioning and, 111–13
sound, sounds, xviii–xix, xxiv, 44, 57, 59, 65, 82–83, 87, 89, 130
soups, soup, 151–54, 163
 butternut squash apple soup, 151
 butternut squash soup, 154
 mung lentil rice soup, 152, 154
spiraling, 159–67, 170
 ancient rituals and, xxxi–xxxii, 159, 162, 164–67
 glowing skin and, 162–63
 haiku poem and, 166–67
 rejuvenating bath and, 164–65
stress, xiii–xiv, xxxii, 2–3, 165
 hidden, xiv, 169–72
 noticing flows and, 140–41
 sensing and, 49, 57
 shifting and, 95, 98, 170, 172
 zoning and, 63, 65, 81
stretching, 21, 31, 75, 95, 144, 154
 grounding and, 13–15
 routines and, 121–23

T

teas, xviii, xxx
 basic detox tea, 150
 cumin coriander fennel (CCF) tea break, 114–15
 herbal teas, 108, 140, 145, 152, 154–55, 163

liver rejuvenation and,
150–51, 154–55
noticing flows and, 140,
142–45
transitioning and, 108–9,
113–15
technology, xxiv, xxix, 57
noticing flows and, 134–36,
138–39
tongue, xviii–xix, 80, 103
tongue IQ, 46–47
tongue scraping, 47, 94,
100–101
**transitioning, xxxi–xxxii,
106–17**
ancient rituals and, xxxii,
108–12, 114, 116
break | fast and, 108–9
cumin coriander fennel
(CCF) tea break and,
114–15
and preparing pot of *khichdi*,
110–11

silence is golden and, 116–17
stress and, 170–71
warm golden milk and, 112–13
Twain, Mark, 37, 140

V

van Gogh, Vincent, 6
Vanzant, Iyanla, 67
vegetables, 47, 97, 172
liver rejuvenation and, 149,
151, 153
transitioning and, 110–11, 114,
116
Vezzani-Katano, Lina, 42
visualizing, xxiv, 9, 127
zoning and, 66, 68, 70, 72, 74,
76, 78

W

Wadsworth, William, 138
walks, 19, 33, 44, 159, 172
nature walk, 44, 130–31
Weekes, Julia, 87

West, Mae, 46
Wilson, Robert Anton, 83
Woolf, Virginia, 111

Z

zones, zoning, xxx, 63–89, 170
ancient rituals and, xxxii,
63–64, 66, 68, 70–72, 74, 76,
78, 80–85, 88–89
blue or B-zone,
74–75, 82
"Good Vibe Poem" and,
82–83
green or G-zone, 72–73, 82
indigo or I-zone,
76–77, 82
judge-free zone, 88–89
orange or O-zone, 68–69, 82
quiet zone, 80–81
red or R-zone, 66–67, 82
re-zone, 84–85
violet or V-zone, 78–79, 82
yellow or Y-zone, 70–71, 82